Anti-Inflammatory Diet Instant Pot Cookbook

Easy Instant Pot Recipes to Decrease Inflammation
Heal Your Body and Lose Weight with Your Electric Pressure Cooker

Anti-Inflammation Meal Plan for Beginners

Tiffany Shelton

Copyright © 2019 by Tiffany Shelton.

All rights reserved.

No part of this book may be reproduced in any form or by any electronic or mechanical means, except in the case of a brief quotation embodied in articles or reviews, without written permission from its publisher.

Disclaimer

The recipes and information in this book are provided for educational purposes only. Please always consult a licensed professional before making changes to your lifestyle or diet. The author and publisher shall have neither liability nor responsibility to anyone with respect to any loss or damage caused or alleged to be caused directly or indirectly by the information contained in this book. All trademarks and brands within this book are for clarifying purposes only and are owned by the owners themselves, not affiliated with this document.

Images from shutterstock.com

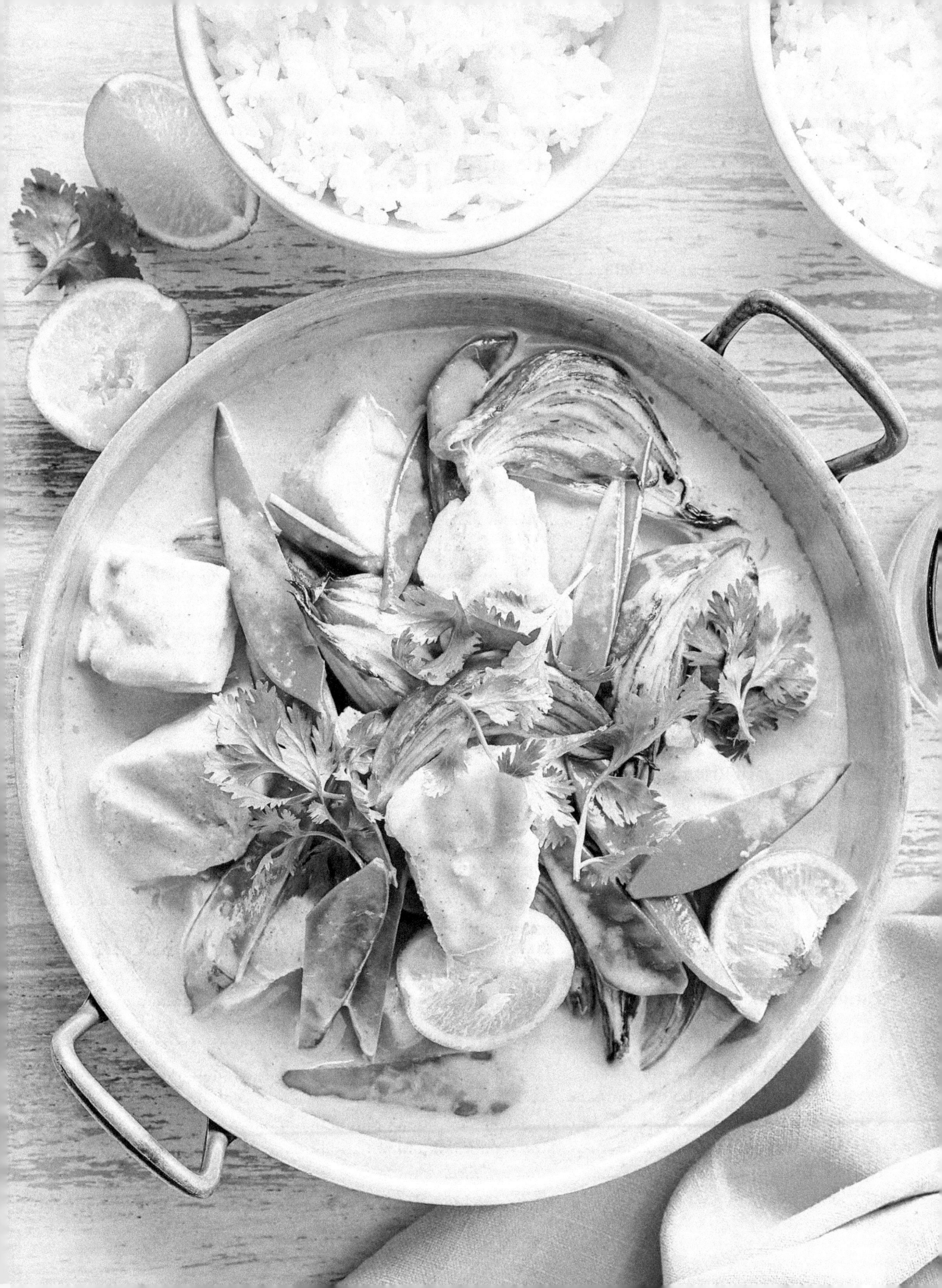

CONTENTS

INTRODUCTION 6

CHAPTER 1. Instant Pot Guide 7

CHAPTER 2. Two-Week Anti-Inflammation Meal Plan 11

CHAPTER 3. Recipes 13

BREAKFAST 13

Pumpkin Flavored Steel Cut Oats 13
Instant Strawberry Jam 14
Cozy Spiced Fruit 15
Maple Brown Sugar Oatmeal 16
20-Minute Steel Cut Oats 17
Pumpkin Pie Oatmeal 18
Coconut Matcha Quinoa 19
Low-Sugar Pineapple Jam 20

LUNCH 21

Tuna Salad 21
Chickpeas & Lentil Salad 22
Green Beans in Mushroom Soup 23
Brown Lentils & Spinach Soup 24
Campfire Baked Beans 25
Coriander Crusted Salmon & Asparagus Salad 26
Creamy Tomato Soup 27
Parsley & Lemon Chickpeas 28
Indian-Style Lentils 29
Risotto Milanese 30
Butternut Squash Risotto 31
Brown Rice & Vegetable Pilaf 32
Basic Bulgur 33

SIDES & SNACKS 34

Herbed Street Corn 34
Less-Salt BBQ Baked Beans 35
Honey-Glazed Carrots 36
Baby Carrots & Mint 37
Parmesan Garlic Artichokes 38

MAIN DISHES 39

Split Pea Soup with Ham 39
Winter Squash & Lentil Stew 40
Chicken Cacciatore 41
Tex-Mex Beef Sammies 42
Apricot-Braised Lamb Shanks 43
Chicken Fricassee 44

Lemon Garlic Chicken 45
Spiced Chicken, Chickpeas & Peppers 46
Chicken in Kale Wraps 47
Chicken with Pesto 48
Beef Casserole 49
Beef with Artichokes 50
Beef with Olives & Feta 51
Beef on Grilled Eggplant 52
Salmon with Tahini Lemon Sauce 53
Greek Vegetable Soup 54
Shrimp, Basil & Spinach Pasta 55
Flounder in Stewed Tomatoes 56
Tomato & Onion Salad with Tofu 57
Broccoli in Lemon Garlic Vinaigrette 58
Collard Greens with Garlic & Bacon 59

DESSERTS 60

Fresh Apple Crumble 60
Brown Rice Pudding 61
Creamy Coconut-Ginger Pudding 62
Cinnamon-Spiked Rice Pudding 63
Warm Spiced Cider 64
Poached Cinnamon Pears 65

CONCLUSION 66

Recipe Index 67

Conversion Tables 68

Other Books by Tiffany Shelton 69

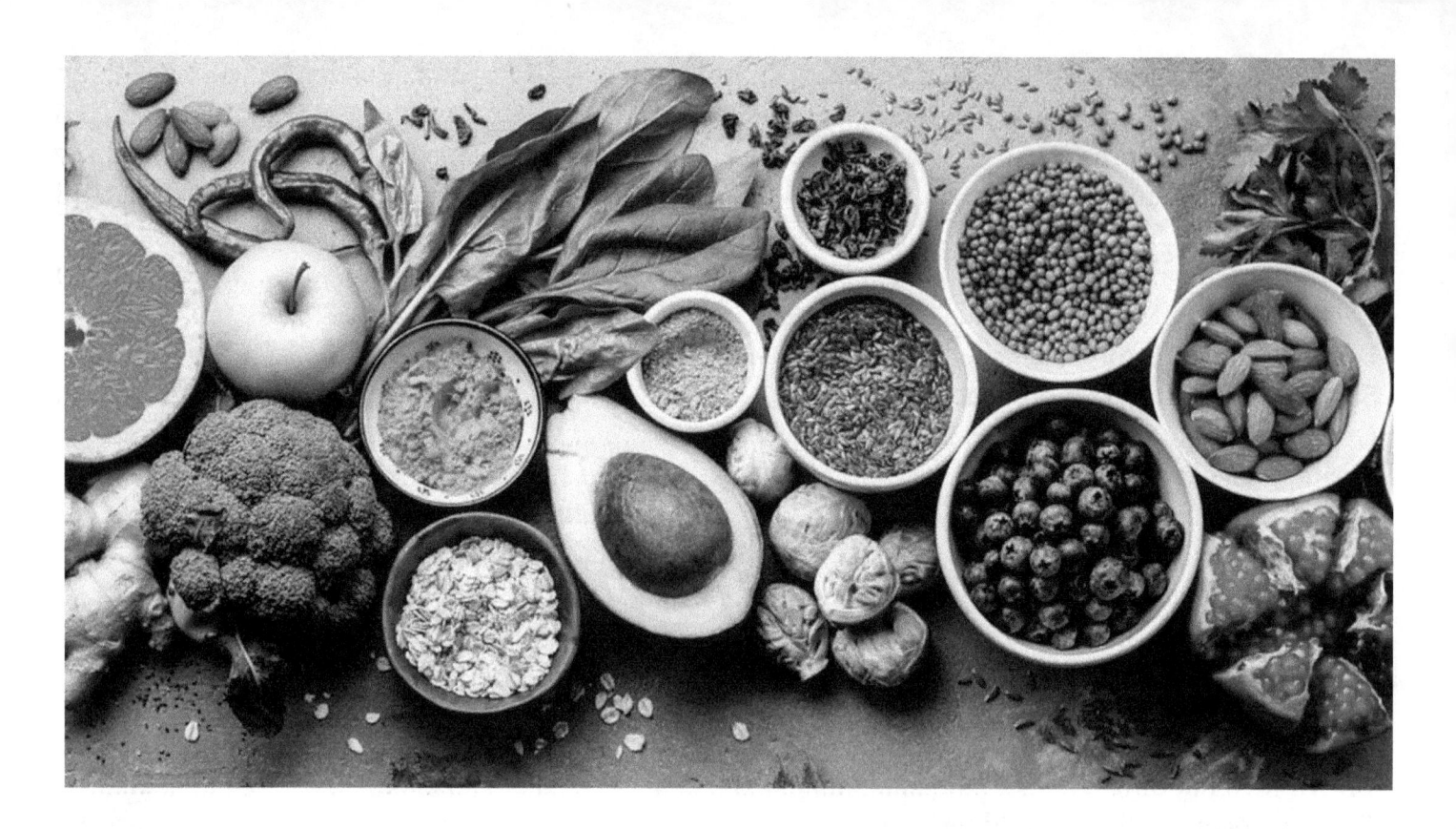

INTRODUCTION

Inflammation is a growing problem worldwide, mainly because poor nutrition, environmental toxins, stress, and limited physical activity have become problems in our society. However, when educated and prepared, you can take control of your health, both preventing inflammation from happening or managing it when it occurs.

From there, you can start on your journey toward an anti-inflammatory diet. The first things that will help you are a simple shopping list, an open mind, and recipes. When it comes to cooking, it's all about getting creative. That's where Instant Pot comes in.

Let's face it, we all struggle to eat healthy, nutritious meals on busy weeknights. When you just have to get food on the table, it's easy to fall back on takeout, frozen meals, and other packaged convenience foods. That can add up quickly when you're on a budget, and this way of eating typically leaves us feeling not so great. That's why so many people love the Instant Pot. It makes healthy cooking easier, so you can enjoy nutritious, homemade meals on a regular basis.

With an Instant Pot, fast and flavorful dishes are within reach no matter how hectic life gets. The quick-cooking power of the Instant Pot means there's no need to spend hours in your kitchen hovering over the stove. And because pressure cooking has proven to be one of the best options available for protecting the nutrients in your food, the Instant Pot is an ideal way to make healthy eating achievable.

CHAPTER 1. Instant Pot Guide

If you've never used Instant Pot before, here's what you need to know to get started right away.

Make sure the stainless-steel insert is clean and properly placed.

Wipe the outside of the stainless-steel pot with a dry towel to make sure nothing has stuck to the bottom or sides after you have placed it on the counter or in the sink. Stuck-on food or debris can interfere with the functioning of your pot, so make sure it's clean each time you use it.

Check that the silicone sealing ring is properly seated in the lid.

The silicone sealing ring expands from the heat and may move around when you take off the lid. Before securing the lid, use your fingers to gently wiggle the sealing ring all around the metal lid to ensure it is properly placed.

Make sure nothing is clogging the vent in your lid.

The stainless-steel cover over the vent is removable, so it's a good idea to clean it every now and then, especially after cooking pasta, to ensure no food or residue is blocking the vent.

Don't overfill the pot.

When cooking foods that are prone to foamings, such as beans or pasta, never fill the pot more than half full and always allow the pressure to naturally release as directed, so the foam doesn't spew out of the release vent. For other recipes, don't fill the pot more than two-thirds full.

Don't preheat the pot.

Although some people preheat the Instant Pot or start with very hot water to reduce the overall cooking time, the recipes in this book assume you are using cool water straight from your faucet or refrigerator. Cooking for less time than the recipes call for may result in your food not cooking as intended.

Don't place your pot directly underneath your kitchen cabinets.

In many cases, you'll need to manually release the steam pressure, which will shoot steam from the top of the pot. Be sure your Instant Pot is situated on a counter with nothing above it, so the hot steam doesn't do any damage.

Unplug your machine when you're done using it.

The Instant Pot goes into an automatic Keep Warm mode when the cooking cycle is complete, which is handy if you're not ready to serve yet. Be sure to unplug the device when you're done using it as a safety precaution.

Now that we've got that covered, here's how to:

Sauté.

The Instant Pot is unique in its ability to also sauté food. This means you can brown meat or sauté vegetables in the pot and then pressure cook in the same pot, or simmer excess liquid out of your sauce when the cooking cycle is over. To use the sauté function, simply press the Sauté button and wait for the beep that tells you the machine is on. Wait for 1 to 2 minutes after the beep for the surface to heat up before you add ingredients to the pot, or they may stick to the bottom. Do not use the lid when using this function; the lid should only be used when pressure cooking.

Cook on Manual.

Press the Manual or Pressure button, depending on your machine, then use the – or + buttons to set the appropriate cooking time. The Manual mode automatically cooks using high pressure, unless you press the Pressure button to switch to low pressure. When pressure cooking, always make sure the steam release valve is moved to the Sealing position. If your machine doesn't have a Manual setting, it most likely cooks on high pressure automatically.

Make sure the pressure has been reached.

There is a floating valve located on the lid next to the steam release valve that pops up when the pot has come to pressure. It usually takes anywhere from 5 to 20 minutes for the valve to pop up, depending on the recipe, and that's when the cooking cycle will begin counting down. Keep an eye on your Instant Pot until the floating valve has popped up to make sure your meal is cooking properly before walking away. You'll hear steam coming out of the vent shortly before the floating valve pops up.

Quickly release the pressure.

To avoid overcooking, many recipes require that you quickly release the pressure as soon as the Instant Pot has beeped to signal the end of a cooking cycle. To do that, carefully move the steam release valve to Venting, keeping your hand away from the top of the vent, so you don't get burned by the steam. As soon as the floating valve drops, remove the lid to stop the cooking process.

Naturally release the pressure.

Allow the lid to remain on the Instant Pot after the cooking cycle has ended until the specified time has passed. Once the cooking cycle has counted down, the timer will start again, counting *up* the minutes to let you know how long it's been since the cooking cycle stopped. If a recipe requires that you let the pressure naturally release for 10 minutes, don't touch the lid until your Instant Pot reads L0:10, which means it has been on a "keep warm" setting for 10 minutes. When the time has passed, move the steam release valve to the Venting position to release any remaining steam before you remove the lid.

Know that it's safe to remove the lid.

After using a quick or natural release and venting any remaining steam in the pot, the floating valve on the lid, which is next to the steam release valve, will drop, letting you know that all of the pressure has been released. The lid has a safety feature that won't let you open it until the valve has dropped.

Use the pot-in-pot cooking method.

This refers to cooking two dishes at the same time, using a separate bowl that fits inside the Instant Pot. To use this time-saving method, you'll need a 2.5-inch trivet and a 7-inch oven-safe bowl that is placed on the trivet over the main entrée, which is cooked directly on the bottom of the Instant Pot. Both the main entrée and the side dish need to cook a similar amount of time for best results.

Cook for 0 (zero) minutes.

Though it might sound strange, some recipes require that you set the pressure cooking cycle for 0 (zero) minutes to ensure that you don't overcook your ingredients. This cooking cycle simply brings the pot to pressure, which can take anywhere from 5 to 20 minutes, and when it beeps and displays L0:00 on the screen, you quickly release the pressure by moving the steam release valve to Venting. Releasing the pressure can take 1 to 2 minutes more, so the food will be sufficiently cooked despite the short cooking time.

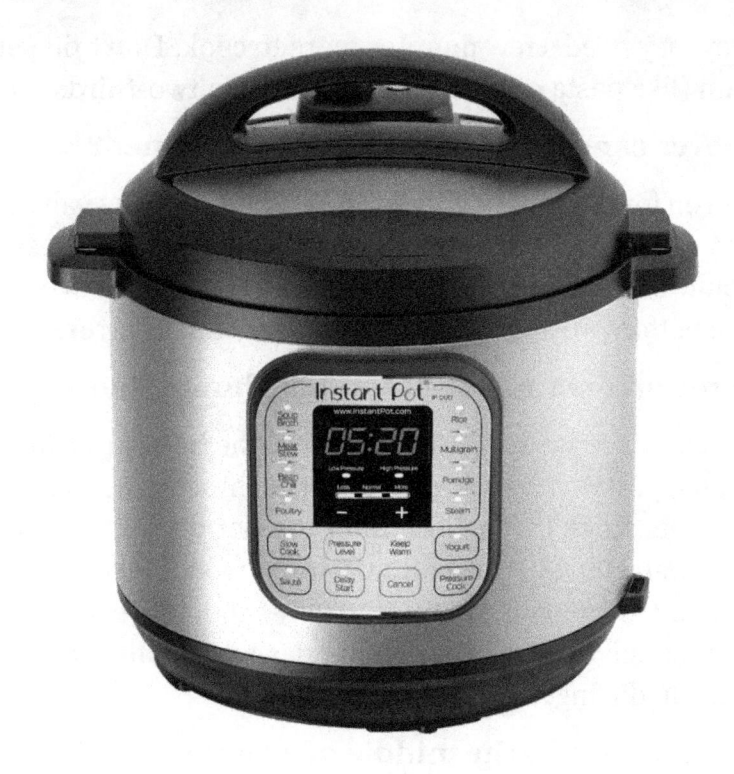

If you run into problems, the following tips should help:

- ✓ **I've selected the cooking program, but my pot just says "on." Why hasn't the countdown started yet?**

After you select your cooking program and cooking time, the Instant Pot waits 10 seconds to start. When it beeps, you'll see an "On" message as it starts to come to pressure. The cooking cycle won't start counting down until the pot is pressurized, and that process can take anywhere from 5 to 20 minutes after you set the timer, depending on how much liquid is in the pot. The less liquid, the faster it will come to pressure.

- ✓ **How do I adjust the cooking time and pressure setting?**

After selecting the Manual or Pressure button, use the − and + buttons to adjust the time. The Manual setting cooks at high pressure automatically, but you can press the Pressure button to adjust the pressure to low on certain models.

- ✓ **Will these recipes work for an 8-quart Instant Pot?**

All of these recipes have been successfully tested using the 8-quart Instant Pot Duo. When using this size pot, follow the recipe directions closely, as the 8-quart is prone to displaying "Burn" errors. In any recipe that calls for sautéing meat or vegetables first, always deglaze the pan before bringing the pot to pressure, so nothing sticks to the bottom. You can do this by adding a splash of water to the hot pan, then using a wooden spoon or spatula to scrape the bottom of the pan to remove anything that has stuck. Recipes don't always need a full cup of added liquid to make this model come to pressure, but you do need to make sure the ingredients are layered in the correct order to avoid burn errors. Also, keep in mind that vegetables might lose their crunch when cooked in this pot due to the longer pressurization time.

- ✓ **Do I need to adjust the cooking time if I double the recipe?**

In most cases, you can double a recipe without changing the cooking time, but keep in mind that the increased volume will naturally increase the overall time it takes to prepare the dish because the Instant Pot may take longer to come to pressure. If you're using particularly large cuts of meat, such as large or frozen chicken breasts, they may need a few minutes more to cook. Don't fill your pot more than half full for items that produce foam (like pasta or beans) and more than two-thirds full for everything else.

✓ My Instant Pot never came to pressure. What happened?

If your Instant Pot has been on for more than 25 minutes and the floating valve hasn't popped up to signal that the pressure has been reached, check to make sure you've moved the steam release to Sealing. If that's not the issue, it could be that the sealing ring in the lid has moved and isn't sealing, or that something was stuck to the bottom of your pot, triggering the "Burn" error.

✓ I see a "Burn" error on my Instant Pot. What should I do?

The "Burn" or "Hot" message on the Instant Pot means that the bottom surface of the stainless-steel pot is getting too hot. This can happen when your Instant Pot is empty, when you're heating the pot to sauté something, and when food gets stuck to the bottom of the pot during the cooking process. To remove stuck food, add a splash of water to the hot pan and use a wooden spoon to scrape the bottom until nothing is stuck. The error message will go away quickly, and you can continue with your recipe as directed. Also, be sure that you have moved the steam release valve to Sealing, so the liquid in your pot doesn't evaporate as it heats up during a pressure cooking cycle.

✓ The floating valve dropped in the middle of a cooking cycle. What should I do?

If steam is coming out of your Instant Pot's floating valve *after* the pressure cooking cycle has started counting down, that means the pot is no longer pressurized, and your meal isn't cooking properly. If you can, gently grab the lid by its handle (don't touch the metal as it's very hot) and press down to see if the lid will seal and pop the valve back up. Sometimes, that's all it takes. If the valve doesn't pop up, you'll need to press Cancel, move the steam release valve to Venting to make sure the pressure is fully released, and remove the lid. Add a bit more liquid to the pot, starting with just ¼ cup water if it looks like there is plenty of liquid at the bottom, or using more if it looks like much of the cooking liquid has simmered away. Use a wooden spoon to scrape the bottom of the pot, making sure nothing has stuck, then close the lid, move the steam release valve to Sealing, and start the pressure cooking process again. Use your best judgment on the timing based on how much cooking time was left in the cycle when the pressure was lost.

✓ Steam is coming out around the rim of my lid. What should I do?

If you see steam coming out around the rim of your lid, and not just from the steam release valve, that is a sign that something is wrong with your sealing ring. You'll have to press Cancel, move the steam release valve to Venting to make sure the pressure is fully released, and remove the lid to check the sealing ring. It's not uncommon for the sealing ring to expand from the heat and move out of place, breaking the seal, so you may be able to fix this issue by pushing the ring back into place and sealing the lid again to continue pressure cooking. If the sealing ring appears to be cracked or damaged, you'll need to buy a replacement.

✓ Why won't my Instant Pot open?

The Instant Pot is designed to stay closed as a safety precaution when the pot is coming to pressure, so you can't open it until the floating valve has dropped. Before attempting to remove the lid, remember to move the steam release valve to Venting and wait for all of the steam to release and the floating valve to drop.

Now that we've covered the basics let's get cooking!

CHAPTER 2. Two-Week Anti-Inflammation Meal Plan

Week 1

	Breakfast	Lunch	Snack	Dinner
Monday	Maple Brown Sugar Oatmeal Page 16	Chickpeas & Lentil Salad Page 22	Less-Salt BBQ Baked BeansLess-Salt BBQ Baked Beans Page 35	Winter Squash & Lentil Stew Page 40
Tuesday	20-Minute Steel Cut Oats Page 17	Tuna Salad Page 21	Baby Carrots & Mint Page 37	Chicken Cacciatore Page 41
Wednesday	Pumpkin Pie Oatmeal Page 18	Campfire Baked Beans Page 25	Herbed Street Corn Page 34	Lemon Garlic Chicken Page 45
Thursday	Pumpkin Flavored Steel Cut Oats Page 13	Brown Lentils & Spinach Soup Page 24	Baby Carrots & Mint Page 37	Chicken Fricassee Page 44
Friday	Low-Sugar Pineapple Jam Page 20	Coriander Crusted Salmon & Asparagus Salad Page 26	Parmesan Garlic Artichokes Page 38	Tex-Mex Beef Sammies Page 42
Saturday	Coconut Matcha Quinoa Page 19	Parsley & Lemon Chickpeas Page 28	Honey-Glazed Carrots Page 36	Flounder in Stewed Tomatoes Page 56
Sunday	Low-Sugar Pineapple Jam Page 20	Indian-Style Lentils Page 29	Parmesan Garlic Artichokes Page 38	Apricot-Braised Lamb Shanks Page 43

Week 2

	Breakfast	**Lunch**	**Snack**	**Dinner**
Monday	20-Minute Steel Cut Oats Page 17	Butternut Squash Risotto Page 31	Honey-Glazed Carrots Page 36	Lemon Garlic Chicken Page 45
Tuesday	Maple Brown Sugar Oatmeal Page 16	Basic Bulgur Page 33	Herbed Street Corn Page 34	Salmon with Tahini Lemon Sauce Page 53
Wednesday	Pumpkin Flavored Steel Cut Oats Page 13	Tuna Salad Page 21	Baby Carrots & Mint Page 37	Greek Vegetable Soup Page 54
Thursday	Low-Sugar Pineapple Jam Page 20	Green Beans in Mushroom Soup Page 23	Parmesan Garlic Artichokes Page 38	Tomato & Onion Salad with Tofu Page 57
Friday	Coconut Matcha Quinoa Page 19	Coriander Crusted Salmon & Asparagus Salad Page 26	Honey-Glazed Carrots Page 36	Flounder in Stewed Tomatoes Page 56
Saturday	Low-Sugar Pineapple Jam Page 20	Parsley & Lemon Chickpeas Page 28	Herbed Street Corn Page 34	Apricot-Braised Lamb Shanks Page 43
Sunday	Maple Brown Sugar Oatmeal Page 16	Chickpeas & Lentil Salad Page 22	Less-Salt BBQ Baked BeansLess-Salt BBQ Baked Beans Page 35	Chicken Cacciatore Page 41

CHAPTER 3. Recipes
BREAKFAST

Pumpkin Flavored Steel Cut Oats

Prep time: 5 minutes

Cooking time: 7 minutes

Servings: 4

Nutrients per serving:

Carbohydrates – 49.2 g

Fat – 2.5 g

Protein – 5.4 g

Calories – 228

Ingredients:

- 3 cups whole milk
- ¾ cup steel-cut oats
- ¾ cup canned pumpkin puree
- 2 Tbsp. brown sugar, add more if desired
- 1 tsp. pumpkin spice mix
- ⅓ cup raisins

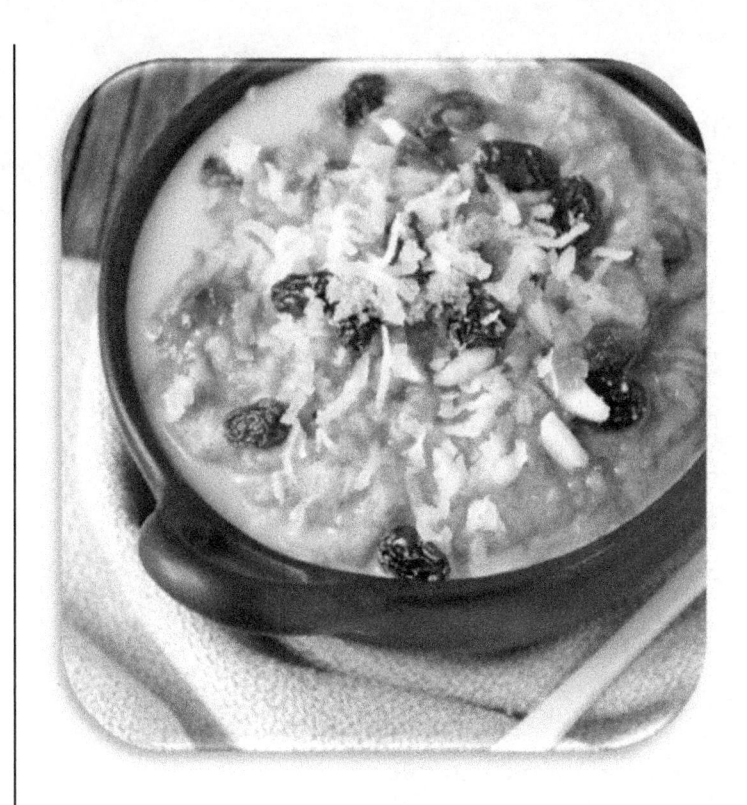

Instructions:

1. Add all ingredients into the Instant Pot, except for pumpkin spice mix and raisins. Stir well.
2. Cover and lock lid. Select Pressure Cook (High). Set cooking time to 7 minutes. After finishing, quick release the pressure.
3. Wait for steam to subside before removing lid. Cool slightly before proceeding.
4. Stir in pumpkin spice mix and raisins. Adjust seasoning, if needed.
5. Serve equal portions of oats in the bowls. Serve.

Instant Strawberry Jam

Prep time: 5 minutes

Cooking time: 36 minutes

Servings: 16 oz

Nutrients per serving:

Carbohydrates – 4 g

Net Carbs – 4 g

Fat – 0 g

Protein – 0 g

Calories – 21

Ingredients:

- 1 pound frozen strawberries
- ¼ cup pure maple syrup
- Pinch of fine sea salt
- 2 Tbsp chia seeds

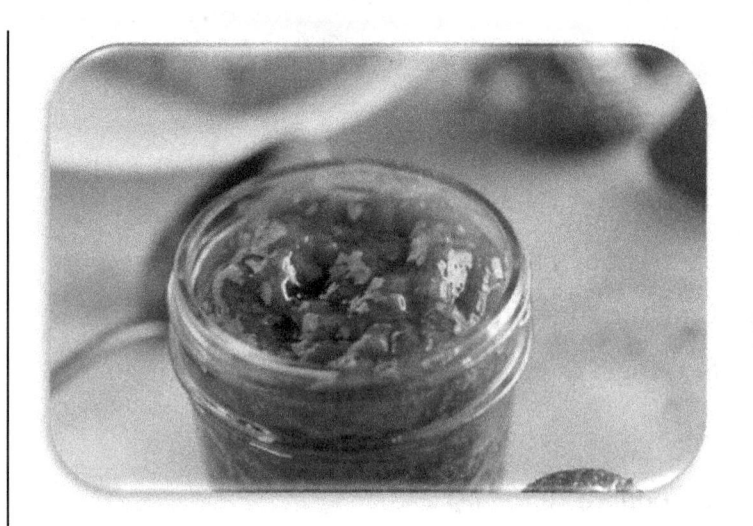

Instructions:

1. Combine the frozen strawberries, maple syrup, and salt in the Instant Pot.
2. Cover and lock lid. Select Manual/Pressure Cook and cook at high pressure for 1 minute.
3. Release the pressure naturally for 10 minutes, then move the steam release valve to Venting. Uncover and press Cancel.
4. Press the Sauté button and add the chia seeds. Simmer the jam until it begins to thicken, about 5 minutes.
5. Once the mixture has thickened slightly, or if the jam starts to stick to the pan, press Cancel to stop the cooking cycle.
6. Let cool. Serve.

Cozy Spiced Fruit

Prep time: 20 minutes

Cooking time: 16 minutes

Servings: 4

Nutrients per serving:

Carbohydrates – 37 g

Fat – 1 g

Protein – 1 g

Calories – 145

Ingredients:

- 1 pound frozen pineapple chunks
- 1 cup frozen and pitted dark sweet cherries
- 2 ripe pears, sliced
- ¼ cup pure maple syrup
- ½ cup almonds, chopped
- 1 tsp curry powder, plus more as needed

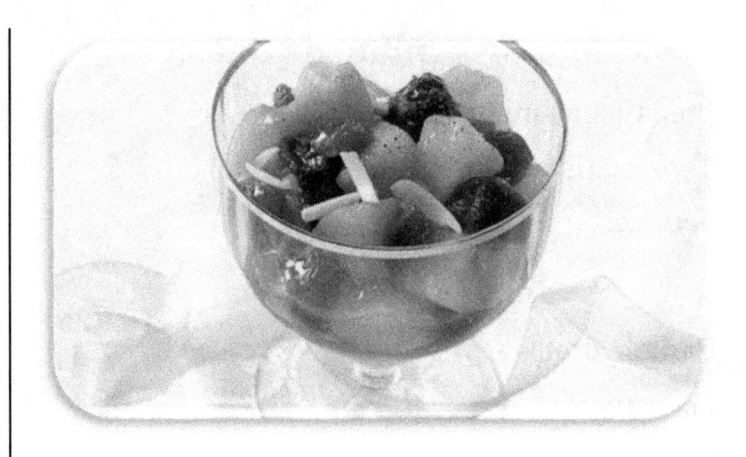

Instructions:

1. Combine all ingredients in the Instant Pot.
2. Cover and lock lid. Select Manual/Pressure Cook and cook at high pressure for 1 minute.
3. When the cooking cycle is complete, quickly move the steam release valve to Venting to release the steam pressure. Uncover and stir the mixture well, adding almonds.
4. It is normal for the fruit to be sitting in its juices when this dish is done. Scoop it with a slotted spoon and let the juices drain back into the pot before serving as a side dish or as a topping for oatmeal.

Maple Brown Sugar Oatmeal

Prep time: 2 minutes

Cooking time: 4 minutes

Servings: 2

Nutrients per serving:

Carbohydrates – 51 g

Fat – 12 g

Protein – 6 g

Calories – 244

Ingredients:

- 1 cup rolled oats
- 1¾ cups water
- Pinch kosher salt
- 1 Tbsp maple syrup
- 2 tsp light brown sugar, lightly packed1 medium banana, sliced

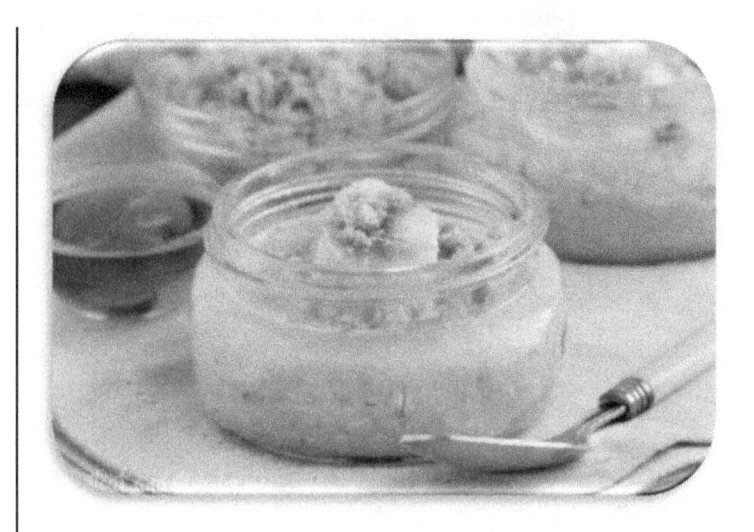

Instructions:

1. Spray the inner pot with nonstick cooking spray.
2. Combine the oats, water, and kosher salt in the pot.
3. Cover and lock lid. Select Pressure Cook (High) and cook time for 4 minutes. After finishing, quick release the pressure.
4. Remove the lid. Add the maple syrup and brown sugar. Stir to combine.
5. Transfer to serving bowls and top each serving with half of the sliced banana.

20-Minute Steel Cut Oats

Prep time: 2 minutes

Cooking time: 10 minutes

Servings: 4

Nutrients per serving:

Carbohydrates – 30 g

Fat – 3 g

Protein – 7 g

Calories – 175

Ingredients:

- 1 cup steel cut oats
- 2½ cups water
- ½ tsp ground cinnamon
- 1 Tbsp light brown sugar
- ¼ tsp kosher salt
- 1 cup fresh strawberries, sliced

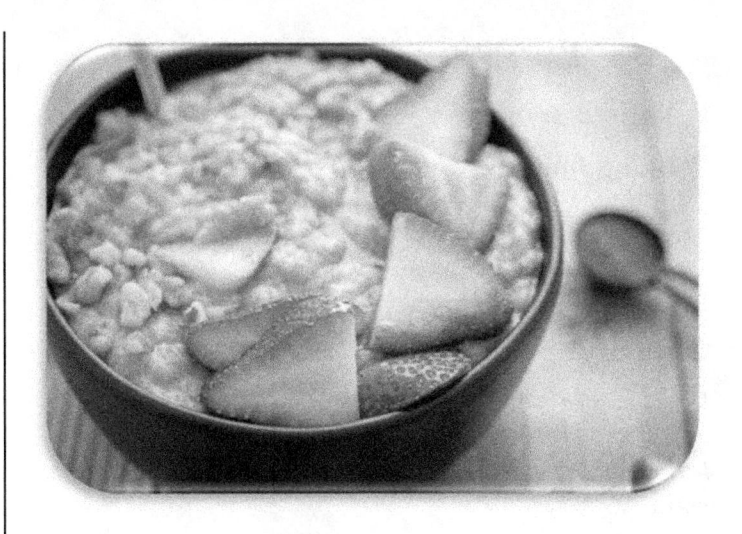

Instructions:

1. Spray the inner pot with nonstick cooking spray.
2. Combine the oats, water, cinnamon, brown sugar, and kosher salt in the pot. Stir well.
3. Cover and lock lid. Select Pressure Cook (High), and cook for 10 minutes. Quick release the pressure.
4. Remove the lid, and allow the oats to cool slightly in the pot. Transfer to serving bowls and garnish each serving with a ¼ cup of the strawberry slices. Serve warm.

Pumpkin Pie Oatmeal

Prep time: 2 minutes

Cooking time: 4 minutes

Servings: 2

Nutrients per serving:

Carbohydrates – 54 g

Fat – 5 g

Protein – 7 g

Calories – 272

Ingredients:

- 1 Tbsp pumpkin seeds
- ½ cup crushed animal crackers
- 1 cup rolled oats
- ¼ cup Pumpkin-Apple Butter
- (see p30)
- 1½ cups water
- Pinch kosher salt

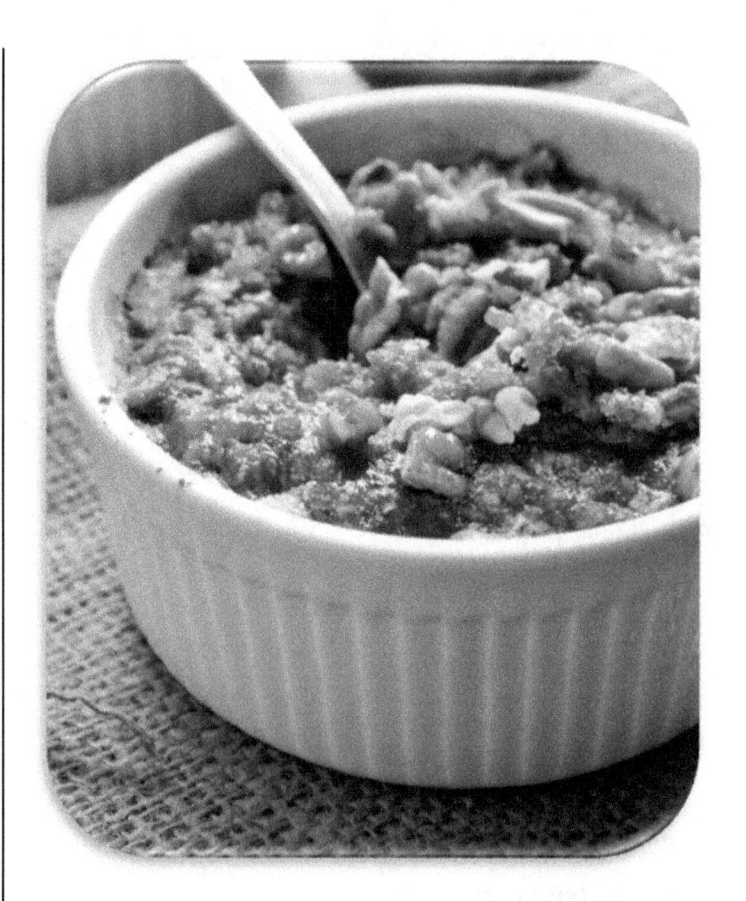

Instructions:

1. Divide the pumpkin seeds and crushed animal crackers into 4 equal-sized portions. Set aside.
2. Spray the inner pot with nonstick cooking spray. Combine the oats, Pumpkin-Apple Butter, water, and kosher salt in the inner pot. Stir well.
3. Cover and lock lid. Select Pressure Cook (High), and set the cook time for 10 minutes. After finishing, quick release the pressure.
4. Remove the lid, and stir. Transfer to serving bowls, and top each serving with the pumpkin seed and animal cracker mix. Serve warm.

Coconut Matcha Quinoa

Prep time: 5 minutes

Cooking time: 15 minutes

Servings: 4

Nutrients per serving:

Carbohydrates – 36 g

Fat – 6 g

Protein – 7 g

Calories – 435

Ingredients:

- 2 Tbsp dried cranberries
- 2 Tbsp roasted pumpkin seeds
- 1 cup quinoa (white or red), rinsed and drained
- ½ cup coconut milk
- ½ cup water
- 1 tsp green tea matcha powder
- 1 Tbsp honey
- Pinch salt

Instructions:

1. Spray the inner pot with nonstick cooking spray.
2. Combine the dried cranberries and pumpkin seeds in a small bowl. Set aside.
3. Combine the quinoa, coconut milk, water, matcha powder, honey, and salt in the inner pot. Stir well.
4. Cover, lock the lid. Select Pressure Cook (High), and cook for 10 minutes. When the cook time is complete, quick release the pressure.
5. Remove the lid, stir, and then transfer to serving bowls. Top each serving with 1 Tbsp of the cranberry and pumpkin seed mixture. Serve warm.

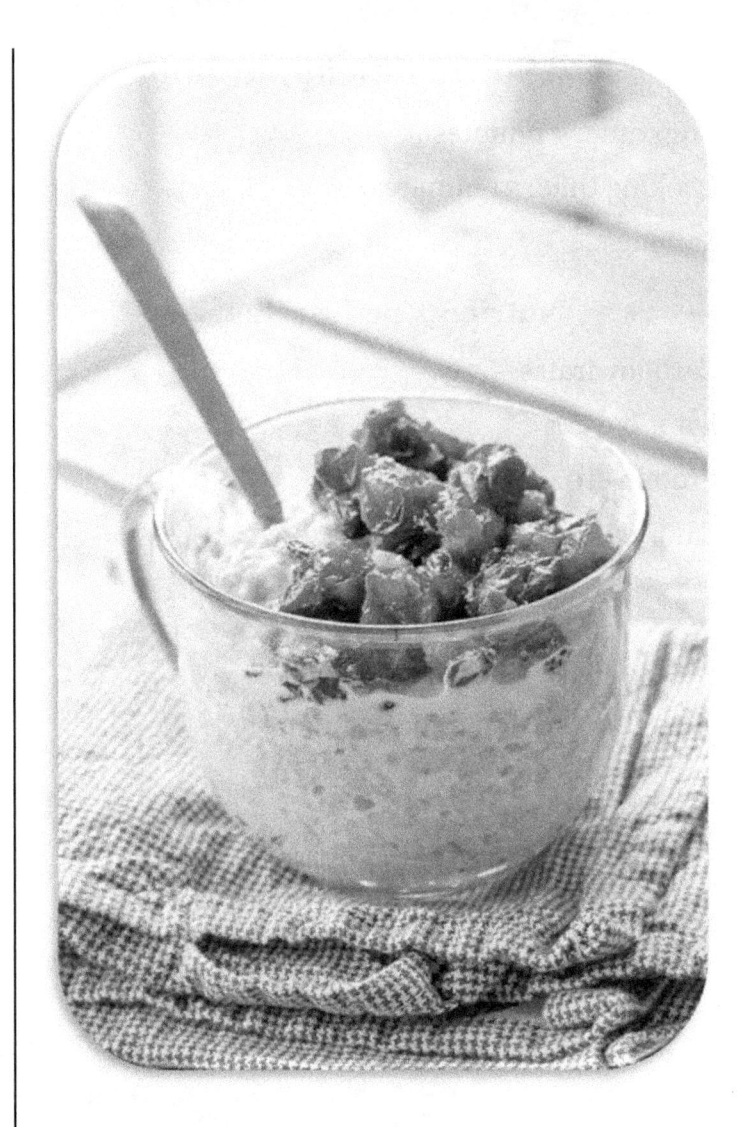

Low-Sugar Pineapple Jam

Prep time: 5 minutes

Cooking time: 31 minutes

Servings: 4

Nutrients per serving:

Carbohydrates – 5 g

Fat – 0 g

Protein – 0 g

Calories – 18

Ingredients:

- 4 cups diced fresh pineapple
- ¼ cup evaporated cane sugar
- Juice of 1 lime

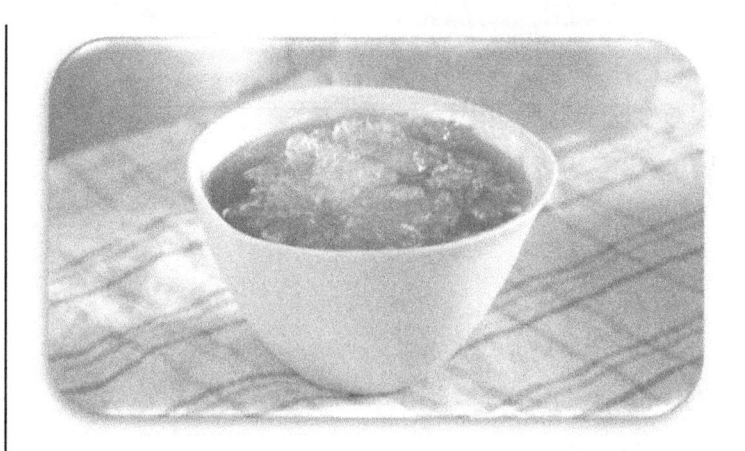

Instructions:

1. Combine ingredients in the inner pot. Stir gently.
2. Cover, lock the lid. Select Pressure Cook (High), and set for 1 minute. Release pressure naturally for about 15 minutes.
3. Remove the lid and stir.
4. If a smoother jam is desired, use an immersion blender to blend the ingredients until a smooth texture is achieved. If a thicker consistency is desired, select Sauté and simmer until the jam thickens, about 10 minutes, and then select Cancel to turn off the heat.
5. Transfer to a large, sealable glass jar and allow to cool completely before sealing.

LUNCH

Tuna Salad

Prep time: 15 minutes

Cooking time: 2 minutes

Servings: 4

Nutrients per serving:

Carbohydrates – 4 g

Fat – 16.3 g

Protein – 9 g

Calories – 189

Ingredients:

- 4 Tbsp olive oil, divided
- 1 Tbsp onion, minced
- 2 cans white albacore tuna, drained
- ½ cup diced roasted red peppers
- 4 Tbsp capers
- 16 Kalamata olives, sliced
- 4 cups lettuce, coarsely chopped
- 2 Tbsp parsley, chopped
- 2 Tbsp lemon juice
- Salt and pepper, to taste

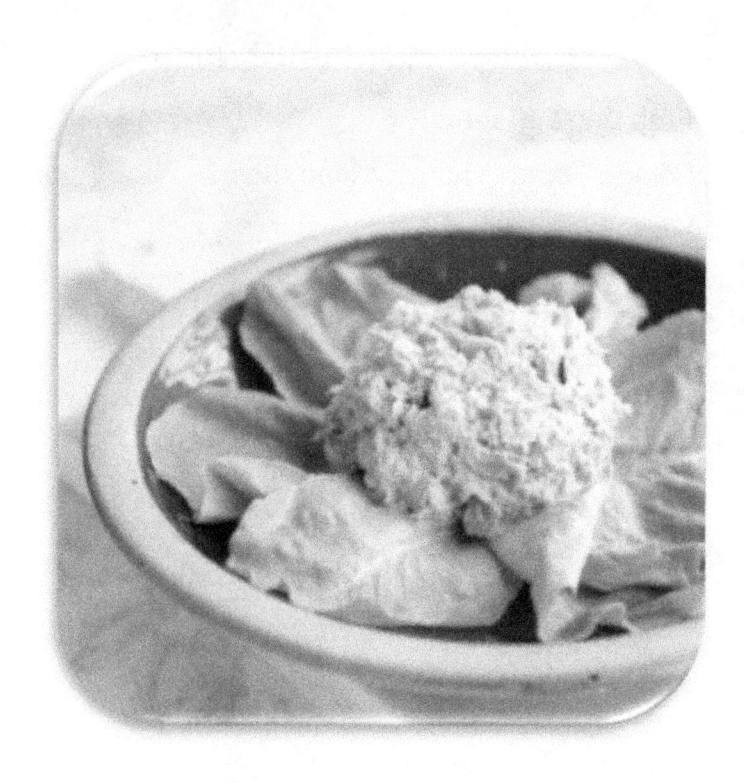

Instructions:

1. Turn your Instant Pot to the Sauté mode.
2. Sauté the onion in 1 Tbsp of olive oil for 2 minutes.
3. Add the tuna and cook for 2 minutes.
4. Add the red peppers, capers, and olives to the mixture.
5. Arrange the lettuce and parsley in a salad bowl, and top with the tuna salad.
6. Drizzle with a mixture of olive oil and lemon juice.
7. Season with the salt and pepper.

Chickpeas & Lentil Salad

Prep time: 20 minutes

Cooking time: 3 hours 43 minutes

Servings: 4

Nutrients per serving:

Carbohydrates – 81 g

Fat – 28.3 g

Protein – 32.9 g

Calories – 702

Ingredients:

- 3 cups water
- 1½ cups dried chickpeas, rinsed
- 1 tsp parsley, chopped
- 1 sprig thyme
- 5 Tbsp olive oil, divided
- 1 cup lentils, rinsed and drained
- 1 tsp Herbes de Provence
- ½ tsp salt
- 1¾ cups vegetable broth
- 4 Tbsp dry white wine, divided
- 1 clove garlic, minced
- ½ cup mint, chopped
- 12 oz cherry tomatoes, quartered
- ¼ cup black olives, chopped
- ½ cup feta cheese, crumbled

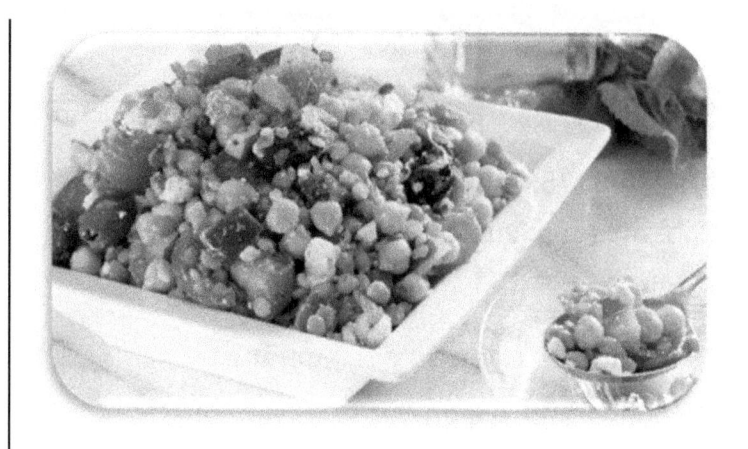

Instructions:

1. Pour the water into the Instant Pot.
2. Add the chickpeas, parsley, thyme, and half of the olive oil. Mix well.
3. Lock the lid in place. Turn to Manual. Cook on high for 38 minutes. Release the pressure naturally.
4. Press the Sauté button. Cook for 5 more minutes, stirring frequently.
5. Drain the chickpeas and set aside. Rinse the pot.
6. Put the chickpeas back with the lentils, Herbes de Provence, salt, broth and half of the white wine. Close the pot. Press the slow cook mode. Cook for 3 hours.
7. In a bowl, mix the garlic, mint, remaining wine, and remaining olive oil.
8. Drizzle the mixture over the lentils and chickpeas.
9. Add the tomatoes and olives.
10. Garnish with the feta cheese before serving.

Green Beans in Mushroom Soup

Prep time: 5 minutes

Cooking time: 20 minutes

Servings: 4

Nutrients per serving:

Carbohydrates – 7 g

Fat – 13 g

Protein – 6 g

Calories – 227

Ingredients:

- 4 slices bacon
- 34 oz frozen green beans
- 2(10.5 oz) cans cream of mushroom soup
- ⅓ cup milk
- 1½ cup fried onions

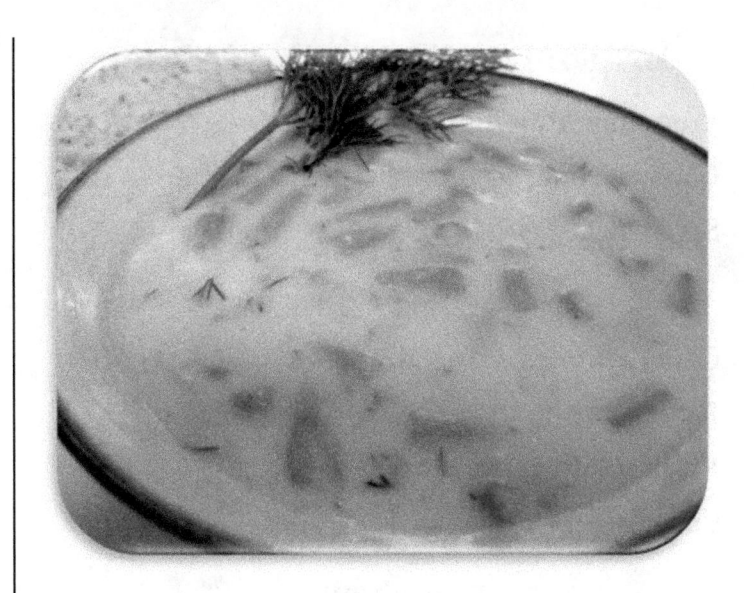

Instructions:

1. Coat your Instant Pot with cooking spray. Set it to the Sauté mode.
2. Cook the bacon slices for 5 minutes. Drain the fat.
3. Add the rest of the ingredients, except the fried onions. Mix well.
4. Seal the pot. Set it to Manual. Cook on low for 15 minutes.
5. Release the pressure Manually.
6. Top with the fried onions before serving.

Brown Lentils & Spinach Soup

Prep time: 10 minutes

Cooking time: 20 minutes

Servings: 4

Nutrients per serving:

Carbohydrates – 20.3 g

Fat – 4.5 g

Protein – 12 g

Calories – 163

Ingredients:

- 2 tsp olive oil
- 1 onion, diced
- 1 stalk celery, diced
- 2 carrots, diced
- 4 cloves garlic, minced
- 1 tsp dried thyme
- 1 tsp ground turmeric
- 2 tsp ground cumin
- Salt and pepper, to taste
- 1 cup brown lentils, rinsed and drained
- 4 cups vegetable broth
- 8 oz baby spinach

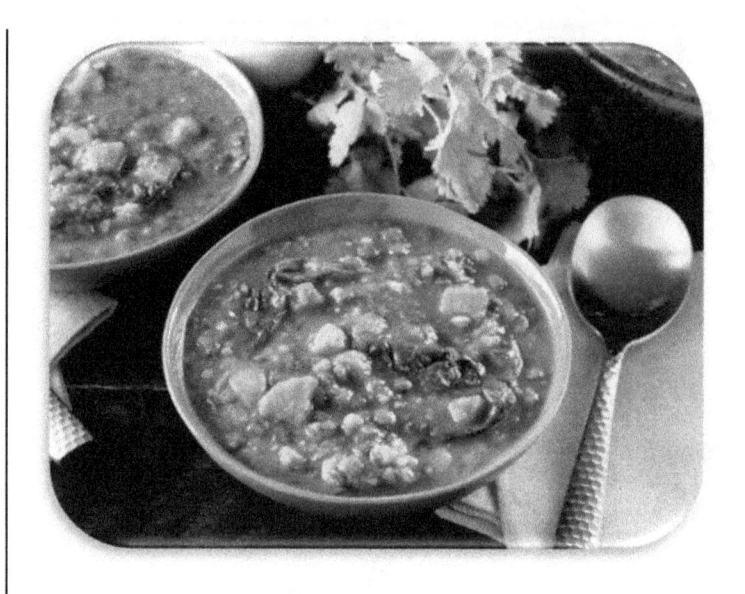

Instructions:

1. Press the sauté button on your Instant Pot. Cook the onion, celery, and carrots for 5 minutes.
2. Add the garlic, thyme, turmeric, cumin, salt, and pepper. Cook for 1 minute.
3. Add the brown lentils and vegetable broth. Stir well. Seal the pot. Choose Manual mode. Cook on high for 12 minutes. Quick release the pressure.
4. Add the spinach and wait for it to wilt before serving.

Campfire Baked Beans

Prep time: 15 minutes

Cooking time: 15 minutes

Servings: 8

Nutrients per serving:

Carbohydrates – 45 g

Fat – 2 g

Protein – 11 g

Calories – 225

Ingredients:

- 1 cup ketchup
- ¼ cup molasses
- 4 tsp mustard powder
- ½ tsp ground black pepper
- 3 slices thick-cut bacon, chopped
- 1 medium onion, chopped
- 1 small green bell pepper, chopped
- 3 15-oz cans lower-sodium navy beans, rinsed and drained
- 2 tsp apple cider vinegar

Instructions:

1. In a bowl, whisk together ketchup, molasses, mustard, and black pepper.
2. In Instant Pot, using Sauté function, cook bacon, onion, and bell pepper, uncovered, for 6 minutes, or until bacon crisps. Hit cancel to turn off Sauté function. Pour off any excess fat.
3. Stir in beans.
4. Spoon ketchup mixture on top; do not stir.
5. Cover and lock lid. Select Manual/Pressure Cook and cook at high pressure for 8 minutes.
6. Once cooking is complete, release pressure by using natural release function. Stir in vinegar and let stand at least 5 minutes for flavors to absorb.

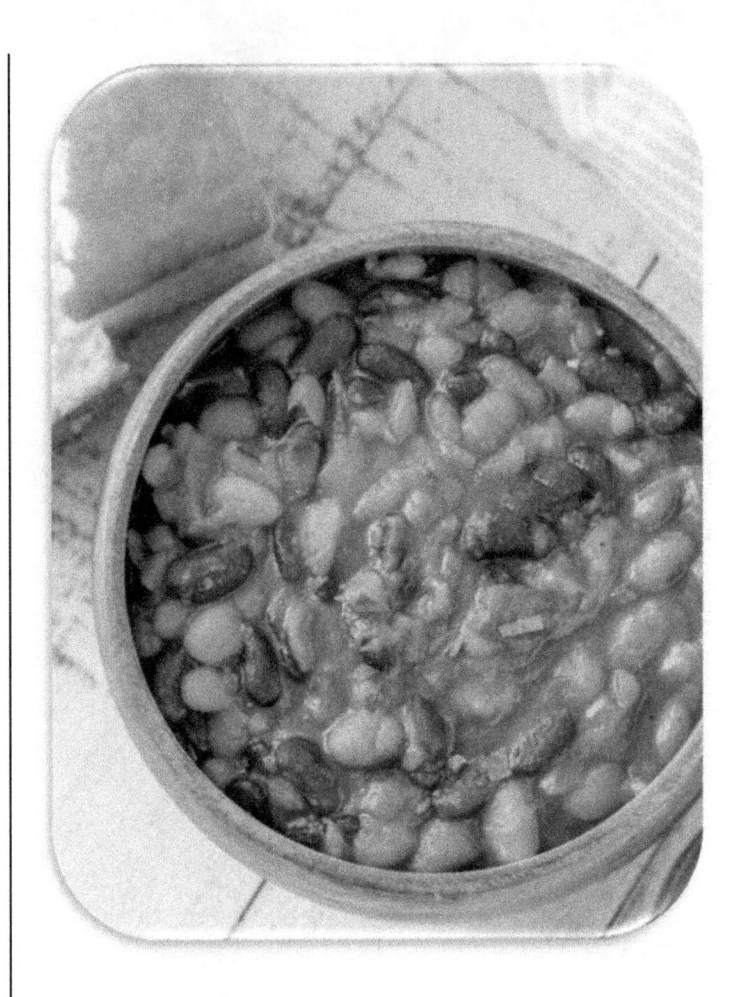

Coriander Crusted Salmon & Asparagus Salad

Prep time: 15 minutes

Cooking time: 3 minutes

Servings: 4

Nutrients per serving:

Carbohydrates – 4 g

Fat – 16 g

Protein – 31 g

Calories – 288

Ingredients:

- 1 tsp lemon zest
- ½ tsp red pepper, crushed
- 1 Tbsp coriander seeds
- ¾ tsp fine sea salt, divided
- 1 lb wild salmon, sliced into 4 portions
- 2 cups water
- 1 lb asparagus, trimmed
- 2 Tbsp olive oil
- 1 Tbsp lemon juice
- 1 Tbsp fresh tarragon, chopped
- 1 Tbsp fresh mint, chopped
- ¼ tsp ground pepper

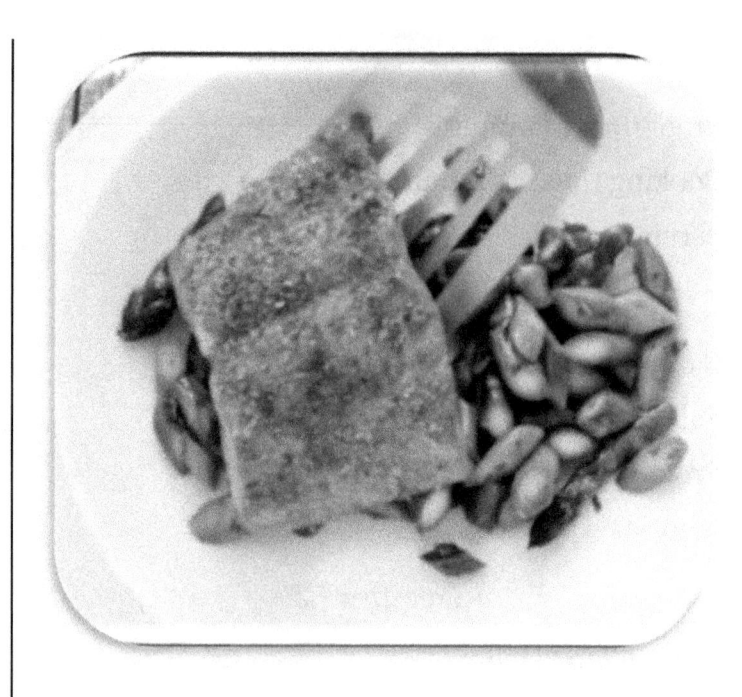

Instructions:

1. Put the lemon zest, red pepper, coriander seeds and ½ tsp salt in a spice grinder. Pulse until finely ground.
2. Cover the salmon with spice mixture.
3. Pour the water into Instant Pot. Place a steamer inside.
4. Place the salmon and asparagus onto the steamer. Close the pot. Set it to Manual. Cook on high for 3 minutes. Release the pressure quickly.
5. In a bowl, mix the olive oil, lemon juice, tarragon, mint, and pepper. Toss the asparagus in this dressing.
6. Serve the salmon with the asparagus salad.

Creamy Tomato Soup

Prep time: 5 minutes

Cooking time: 18 minutes

Servings: 4

Nutrients per serving:

Carbohydrates – 8 g

Fat – 9 g

Protein – 4 g

Calories – 127

Ingredients:

- 12 organic plum tomatoes
- 1 Tbsp olive oil
- 2 cups From-Scratch Chicken Stock (see pg. 100) or low-sodium chicken stock
- 1 clove garlic
- ½ tsp kosher salt
- ¼ tsp freshly ground
- black pepper
- ¼ cup half & half
- 1 cup fresh basil leaves

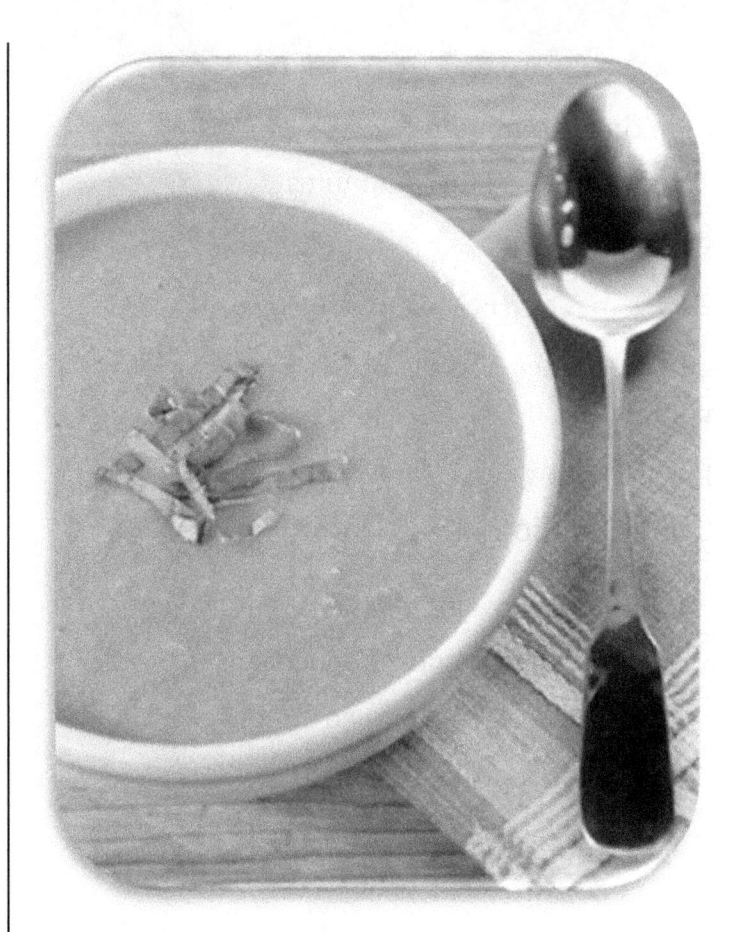

Instructions:

1. Combine the tomatoes, olive oil, chicken stock, garlic clove, kosher salt, and pepper in the inner pot.
2. Cover, lock the lid. Select Pressure Cook (High), and set the cook time for 8 minutes.
3. After finishing, allow the pressure to release naturally for 10 minutes, and then quickly release the remaining pressure.
4. Remove the lid, and add the half & half and basil. Using an immersion blender, purée the ingredients until a smooth consistency is achieved and no lumps remain.
5. Ladle the soup into serving bowls. Serve hot.

Parsley & Lemon Chickpeas

Prep time: 10 minutes

Cooking time: 1 hour 5 minutes

Servings: 4

Nutrients per serving:

Carbohydrates – 33 g

Fat – 13 g

Protein – 10 g

Calories – 280

Ingredients:

- 1 medium onion, chopped
- 1 stalk celery, chopped
- 3 cloves garlic, smashed
- 3 Tbsp olive oil
- 1 cup dried chickpeas
- 1 14.5-oz can lower-sodium chicken broth or 1½ cups homemade chicken broth
- ½ cup water
- 3 Tbsp finely chopped fresh parsley
- ½ tsp grated lemon zest
- 3 Tbsp lemon juice
- ½ tsp salt
- 1 tsp ground black pepper

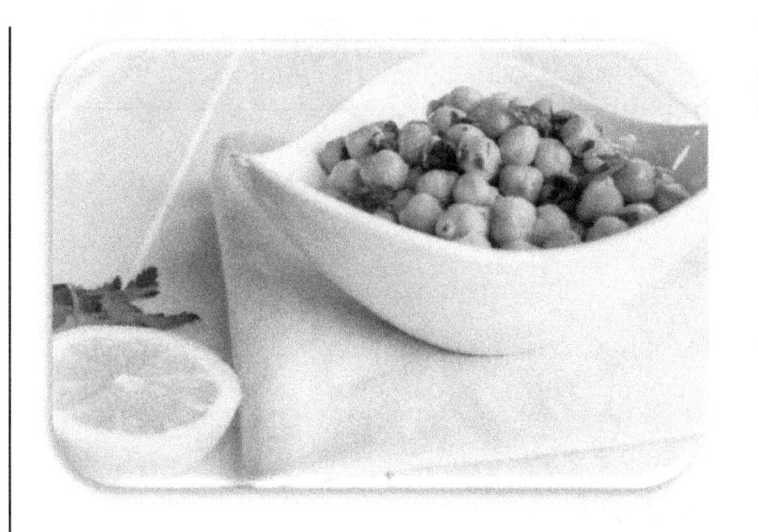

Instructions:

1. In Instant Pot using Sauté function, cook onion, celery, and garlic uncovered, in 1 Tbsp olive oil for 3 minutes, or until softening. Hit cancel to turn off Sauté function.
2. Add chickpeas, broth, and ½ cup water. Cover and lock lid. Select Manual/Pressure Cook and cook at high pressure for 40 minutes.
3. Once cooking is complete, release pressure by using natural release function.
4. Drain chickpeas and discard garlic cloves. Toss in large bowl with parsley, lemon zest, lemon juice, salt, pepper, and remaining 2 Tbsp olive oil.
5. Serve warm or room temperature.

Indian-Style Lentils

Prep time: 15 minutes

Cooking time: 15 minutes

Servings: 6

Nutrients per serving:

Carbohydrates – 38 g

Fat – 4 g

Protein – 12 g

Calories – 225

Ingredients:

- 1 onion, chopped
- 1 Tbsp vegetable oil
- 1 cup brown lentils, rinsed and picked over
- 1 large clove garlic, chopped
- 1½ tsp cumin seeds
- ¼ tsp cayenne pepper
- 1 14.5-oz can chicken or vegetable broth or 1½ cups homemade chicken broth
- ¼ cup water
- 2 Tbsp chopped peeled fresh ginger
- 1 pound sweet potatoes, peeled and cut into ½-inch pieces (about 3 cups)
- ½ tsp salt
- 1 8-oz container plain low-fat yogurt
- ¼ cup chopped fresh mint

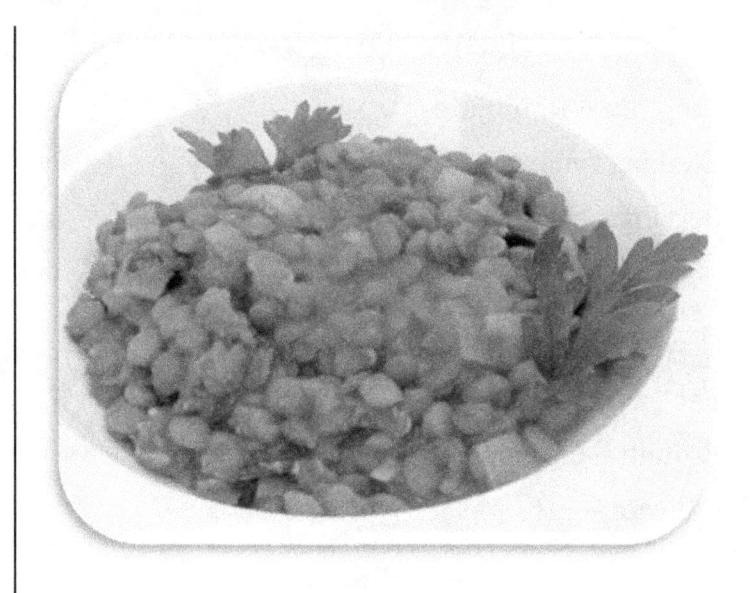

Instructions:

1. In Instant Pot using Sauté function, cook onion in oil, uncovered, for 3 minutes, or until softened. Hit cancel to turn off Saute function.
2. Add lentils, garlic, cumin seeds, cayenne, broth, and ¼ cup water. Cover and lock lid. Select Manual/Pressure Cook and cook at high pressure for 7 minutes.
3. Once cooking is complete, release pressure by using a quick release.
4. Add ginger and sweet potatoes. Cover and lock lid. Select Manual/Pressure Cook and cook at high pressure for 6 minutes.
5. Once cooking is complete, release pressure by using a quick release. Stir in salt. Transfer to serving bowl.
6. In a small bowl, combine yogurt and mint. Serve with lentils.

Risotto Milanese

Prep time: 10 minutes
Cooking time: 20 minutes
Servings: 6

Nutrients per serving:

Carbohydrates – 35 g

Fat – 6 g

Protein – 6 g

Calories – 216

Ingredients:

- 1 medium onion, finely chopped
- 2 Tbsp butter or olive oil
- 2 cups Arborio rice or medium-grain rice
- ½ cup dry white wine
- 1 14.5-oz can chicken broth
- ¼ tsp loosely packed saffron threads
- 1 tsp salt
- ½ cup freshly grated Parmesan cheese, plus more for serving

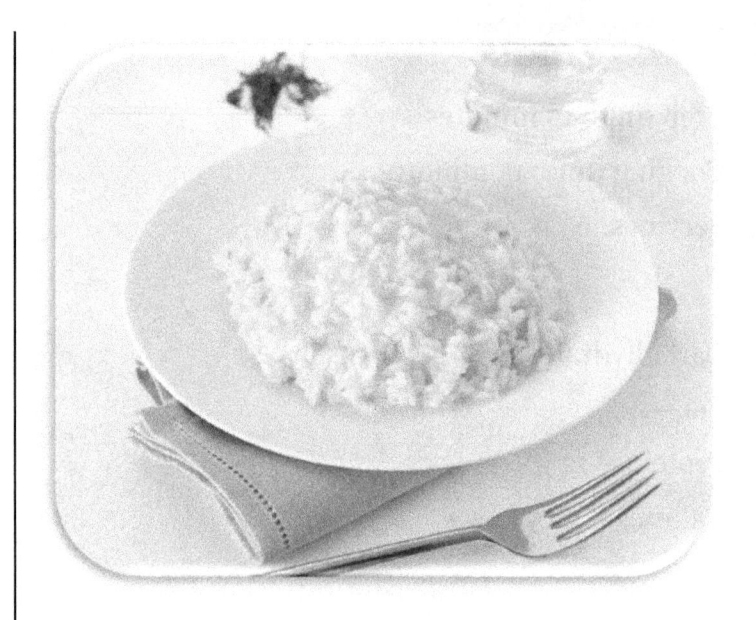

Instructions:

1. In Instant Pot using Sauté function, cook onion in butter, uncovered, for 3 minutes, or until softening.
2. Add rice and stir frequently for 3 minutes, or until grains are opaque.
3. Add wine and cook, stirring, for 1 minute, until absorbed. Hit cancel to turn off Sauté function.
4. Stir in broth, saffron, salt, and 1½ cups water. Cover and lock lid. Select Manual/Pressure Cook and cook at high pressure for 6 minutes.
5. Once cooking is complete, release pressure by using a quick release. Let stand 5 minutes, covered.
6. Stir in Parmesan and add additional ¼ cup water if needed. Serve with grated Parmesan.

Butternut Squash Risotto

Prep time: 15 minutes

Cooking time: 15 minutes

Servings: 4

Nutrients per serving:

Carbohydrates – 91 g

Fat – 7 g

Protein – 11 g

Calories – 465

Ingredients:

- 1 Tbsp olive oil
- 2 medium shallots, chopped
- 3 cloves garlic, finely chopped
- 4 fresh sage leaves, chopped
- ½ tsp salt
- 2 cups Arborio rice
- 4 cups lower-sodium chicken or vegetable broth
- 1 lb butternut squash, cut into ½-inch pieces
- ½ cup freshly grated Parmesan cheese
- ¼ tsp ground black pepper

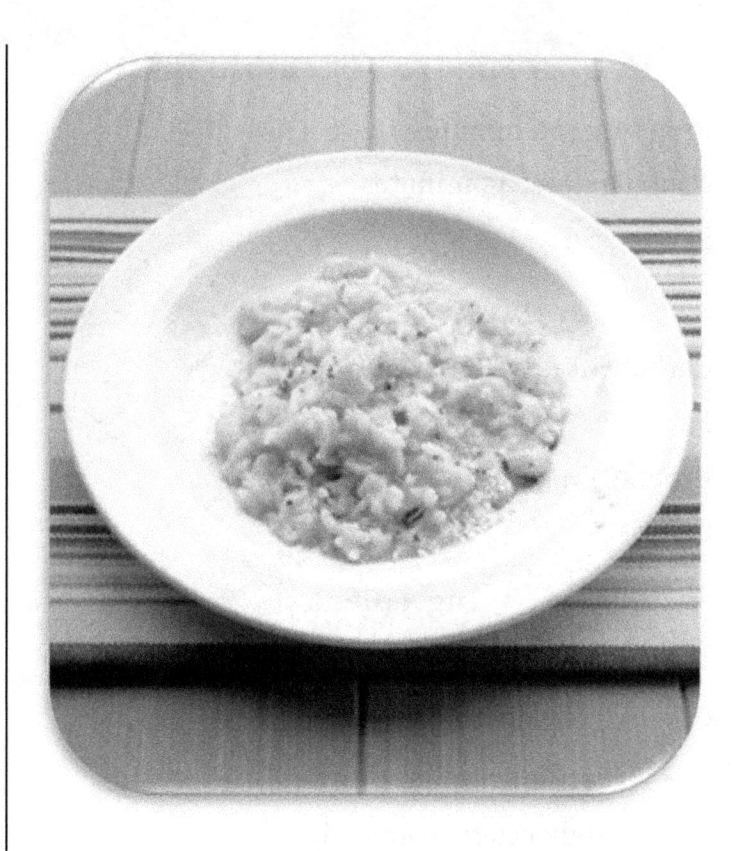

Instructions:

1. In Instant Pot using Sauté function, heat oil. Add shallots, garlic, sage, and ¼ tsp salt. Cook, uncovered, for 2 minutes, stirring.
2. Add rice and cook 2 minutes, stirring. Hit cancel to turn off Sauté function.
3. Add broth and butternut squash. Cover and lock lid. Select Manual/Pressure Cook and cook at high pressure for 6 minutes.
4. Once cooking is complete, release pressure by using a quick release.
5. Stir in Parmesan, remaining ¼ tsp salt, and pepper. Let stand 5 minutes before serving.

Brown Rice & Vegetable Pilaf

Prep time: 10 minutes

Cooking time: 45 minutes

Servings: 6

Nutrients per serving:

Carbohydrates – 31 g

Fat – 3 g

Protein – 4 g

Calories – 67

Ingredients:

- 8 oz cremini mushrooms, sliced
- 1 Tbsp olive or vegetable oil
- 1 medium onion, chopped
- 1 stalk celery, chopped
- 1 cup regular long-grain brown rice
- 2 carrots, chopped
- 1 clove garlic, chopped
- ½ tsp dried thyme
- ¼ tsp dried sage
- 1 Tbsp parmesan
- 1¼ tsp salt
- ¼ tsp ground black pepper

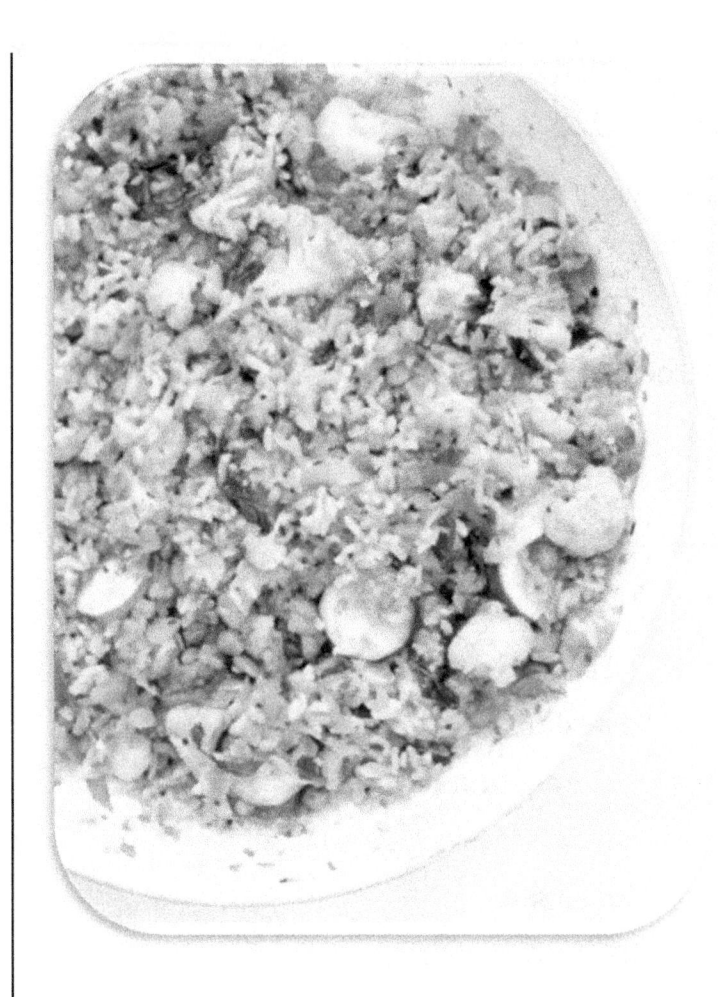

Instructions:

1. In Instant Pot using Sauté function, heat oil. Add shallots, garlic, sage, and ¼ tsp salt. Cook, uncovered, for 2 minutes, stirring.
2. Add rice and cook 2 minutes, stirring. Hit cancel to turn off Sauté function.
3. Add broth and carrots. Cover and lock lid. Select Manual/Pressure Cook and cook at high pressure for 6 minutes.
4. Once cooking is complete, release pressure by using a quick release.
5. Stir in Parmesan, remaining ¼ tsp salt, and pepper. Let stand 5 minutes before serving.

Basic Bulgur

Prep time: 5 minutes

Cooking time: 25 minutes

Servings: 4

Nutrients per serving:

Carbohydrates – 271 g

Fat – 1 g

Protein – 5 g

Calories – 133

Ingredients:

- 1 cup coarse or medium-grind bulgur
- 1 Tbsp canola oil
- 1½ cups chicken broth, store-bought
- ¼ tsp dried thyme
- Pinch of ground nutmeg

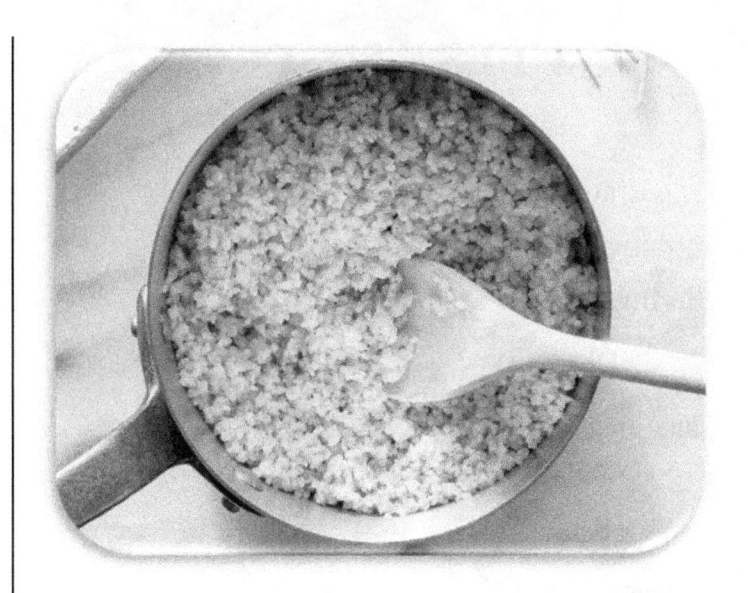

Instructions:

1. In Instant Pot using Sauté function, cook bulgur in oil, uncovered, for 4 minutes, or until fragrantly toasted.
2. Quickly add broth. Stir in thyme and nutmeg. Cover and lock lid. Select Manual/Pressure Cook and cook at high pressure for 6 minutes.
3. Once cooking is complete, release pressure by using natural release function. Let stand 5 minutes and fluff with a fork.

SIDES & SNACKS

Herbed Street Corn

Prep time: 5 minutes

Cooking time: 5 minutes

Servings: 4

Nutrients per serving:

Carbohydrates – 30 g

Fat – 4 g

Protein – 5 g

Calories – 154

Ingredients:

- 4 medium ears corn, shucked
- 4 tsp nonfat Greek yogurt
- 2 tsp mayonnaise
- ¼ tsp kosher salt
- ¼ tsp Freshly ground
- Black pepper, to taste
- 2 Tbsp chopped fresh parsley
- ¼ cup crumbled feta cheese

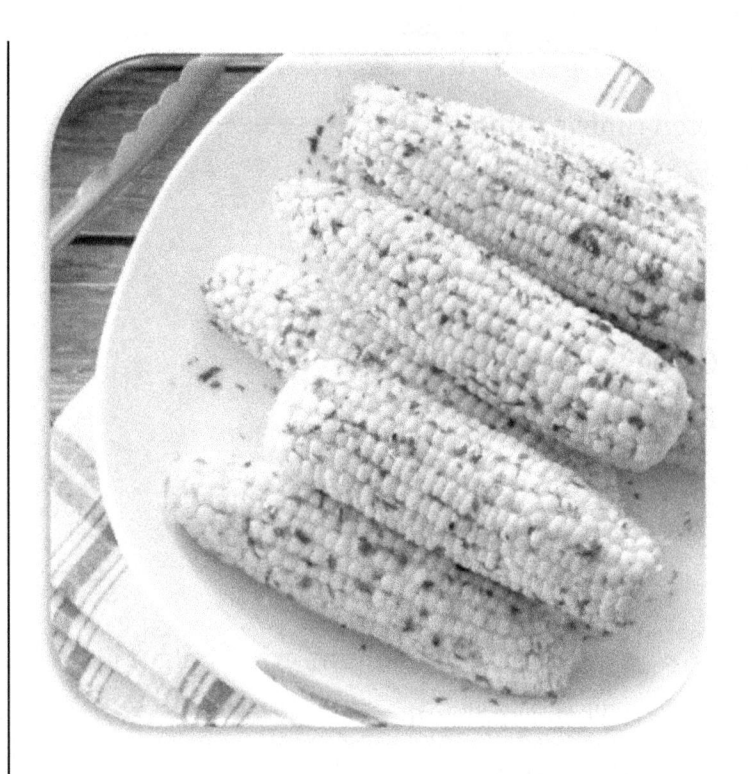

Instructions:

1. Place the steam rack in the inner pot, and add 1 cup water. Place the corn in the pot.
2. Cover, lock the lid. Select Steam (High), adjust the mode to Normal and set the cook time for 5 minutes.
3. Combine the Greek yogurt, mayonnaise, kosher salt, pepper, and parsley in a small bowl. Stir well to mix.
4. When the cook time for the corn is complete, quick release the pressure, remove the lid, and remove the corn.
5. Top each ear with 2 tsp of the sauce, and sprinkle the feta over the top. Serve hot.

Less-Salt BBQ Baked Beans

Prep time: 10 minutes

Cooking time: 4 minutes

Servings: 6

Nutrients per serving:

Carbohydrates – 30 g

Fat – 1 g

Protein – 6 g

Calories – 150

Ingredients:

- 2 Tbsp maple syrup
- 2 Tbsp molasses
- 1 tsp Dijon mustard
- ¼ cup ketchup
- ½ tsp garlic powder
- 2 15-oz cans cannellini or pinto beans, rinsed and drained
- ¼ cup water

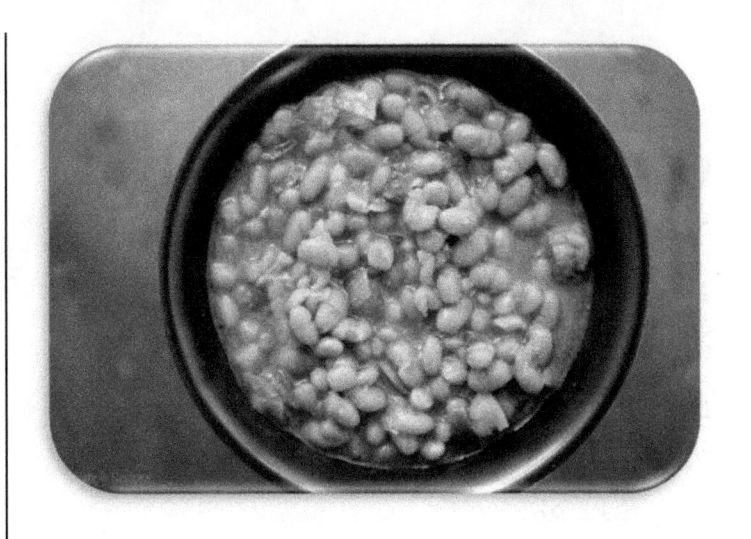

Instructions:

1. Combine the maple syrup, molasses, Dijon mustard, ketchup, and garlic powder in a small bowl. Mix well.
2. Combine the beans, water, and sauce in the inner pot. Mix well to combine.
3. Cover, lock the lid. Select Pressure Cook (Low), and set the cook time for 4 minutes. Quick release the pressure after finished.
4. Remove the lid, stir, and transfer to a serving bowl. Serve hot.

Honey-Glazed Carrots

Prep time: 5 minutes

Cooking time: 10 minutes

Servings: 1

Nutrients per serving:

Carbohydrates – 15 g

Fat – 3 g

Protein – 51 g

Calories – 83

Ingredients:

- 1 lb arrots, peeled and chopped into bite-sized chunks
- 1 cup of water.
- 2 tsp coconut oil
- 1 Tbsp honey
- Kosher salt

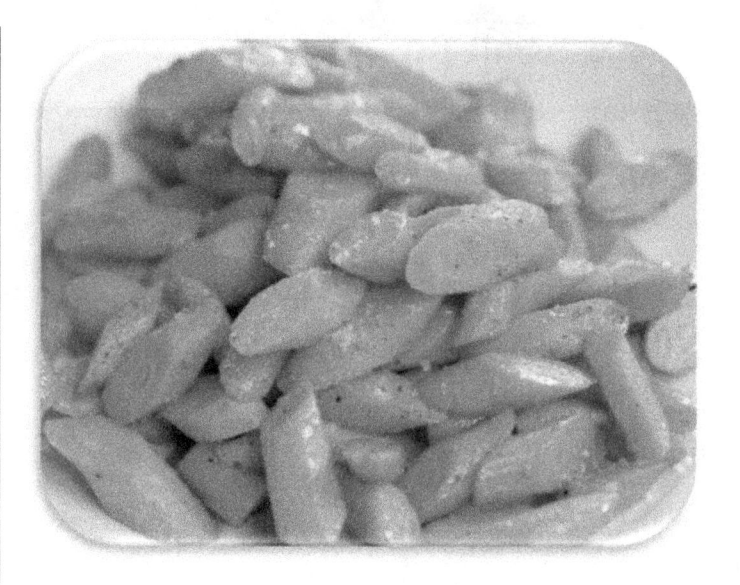

Instructions:

1. Place the steam rack in the inner pot, and add the carrots and 1 cup water.
2. Cover, lock the lid. Flip the steam release handle to the sealing position. Select Steam, and set the cook time for 4 minutes. Quick release the pressure after finishing.
3. Open the lid. Transfer the carrots to a bowl and set aside. Remove the inner pot from the base, drain the water, and return the inner pot to the base.
4. Select Sauté, and add the coconut oil and honey to the inner pot. Heat until the glaze begins to sizzle.
5. Add the cooked carrots back to the pot, and season with a pinch of kosher salt. Toss gently to coat the carrots in the glaze.
6. Transfer to a serving bowl and allow to cool for 5 minutes before serving. Serve warm.

Baby Carrots & Mint

Prep time: 5 minutes

Cooking time: 2 minutes

Servings: 4

Nutrients per serving:

Carbohydrates – 8 g

Fat – 6 g

Protein – 1 g

Calories – 86

Ingredients:

- 4 cups baby carrots
- ½ cup fresh mint, chopped
- 2 Tbsp butter

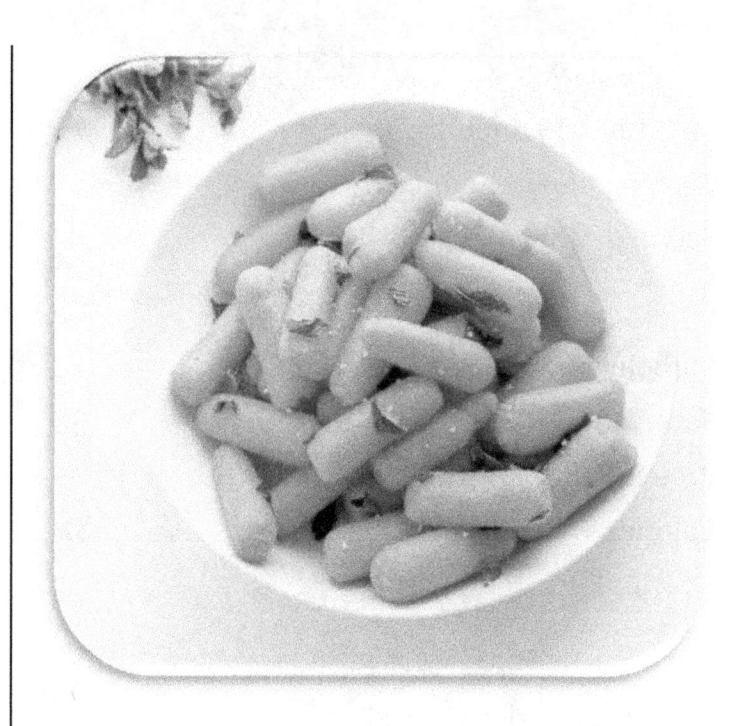

Instructions:

1. Put the carrots inside the Instant Pot.
2. Sprinkle with the fresh mint.
3. Add the butter on top.
4. Seal the pot and turn to Manual.
5. Cook on high for 2 minutes.

Parmesan Garlic Artichokes

Prep time: 10 minutes

Cooking time: 7 minutes

Servings: 4

Nutrients per serving:

Carbohydrates – 17.9 g

Fat – 6.6 g

Protein – 8.3 g

Calories – 146

Ingredients:

- 4 artichokes, washed and trimmed
- 2 tsp garlic, minced
- 4 tsp olive oil
- ¼ cup grated Parmesan cheese
- ½ cup vegetable broth

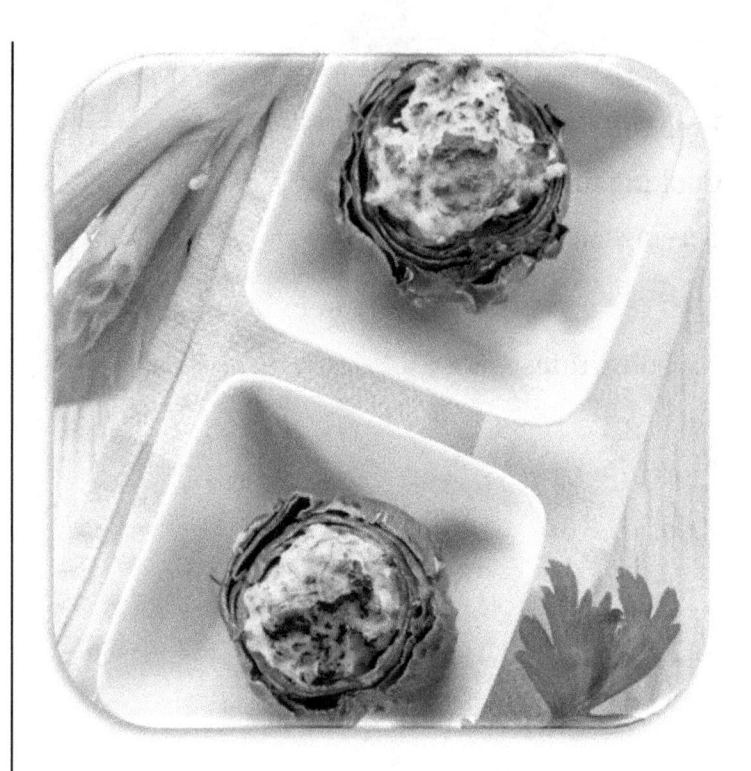

Instructions:

1. Halve the artichokes. Top them with the garlic, olive oil, and Parmesan cheese.
2. Pour the broth into the Instant Pot.
3. Place a steamer basket inside, and put the artichokes on top of the steamer. Cover the pot and choose the steam function. Cook for 7 minutes. Use the quick pressure release method.
4. Let cool and serve.

MAIN DISHES

Split Pea Soup with Ham

Prep time: 10 minutes

Cooking time: 45 minutes

Servings: 3

Nutrients per serving:

Carbohydrates – 54 g

Fat – 14 g

Protein – 29 g

Calories – 455

Ingredients:

- 1 Tbsp vegetable oil
- 1 white turnip, peeled and chopped
- 1 carrot, chopped
- 1 stalk celery, chopped
- 1 medium onion, finely chopped
- 1¼ cups split peas, rinsed and picked over
- 2 smoked ham hocks (1½ pounds total)
- 4 cups water
- 1 bay leaf
- ¼ tsp ground allspice
- ½ tsp salt
- ¼ tsp ground black pepper

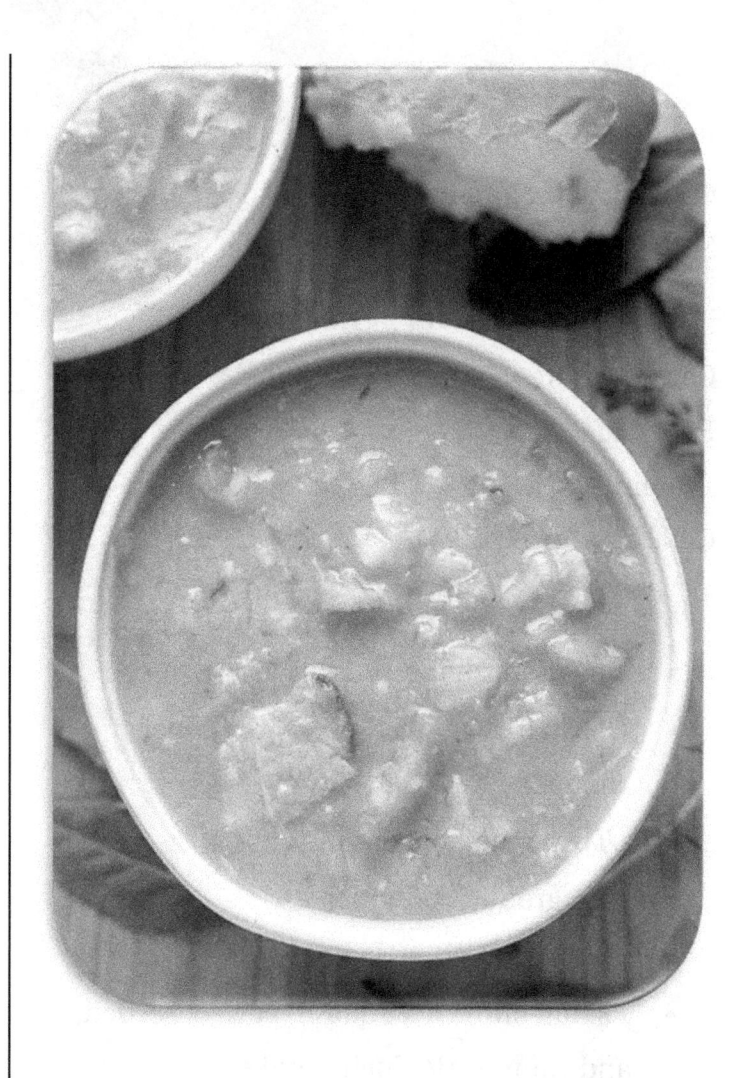

Instructions:

1. In Instant Pot, combine all ingredients.
2. Cover and lock lid. Select Manual/Pressure Cook and cook at high pressure for 8 minutes.
3. Once cooking is complete, release pressure by using natural release function.
4. Discard bay leaf. Transfer ham hocks to cutting board, and discard skin and bones. Finely chop any meat. Stir into soup.

Winter Squash & Lentil Stew

Prep time: 15 minutes

Cooking time: 35 minutes

Servings: 6

Nutrients per serving:

Carbohydrates – 57 g

Fat – 4 g

Protein – 19 g

Calories – 325

Ingredients:

- 2 medium shallots, thinly sliced
- 1 Tbsp fresh ginger, peeled and finely chopped
- 1 Tbsp vegetable oil
- 1 tsp ground coriander
- ½ tsp ground cardamom
- 1 small butternut squash, peeled, seeded, and cut into 1½-inch chunks
- 1 lb green lentils, rinsed and picked over
- 6 cups chicken or vegetable broth, store-bought or homemade (pages 17 and 18)
- Salt, to taste
- 5 cups packed baby spinach
- 1 Tbsp apple cider vinegar
- Freshly ground black pepper, to taste

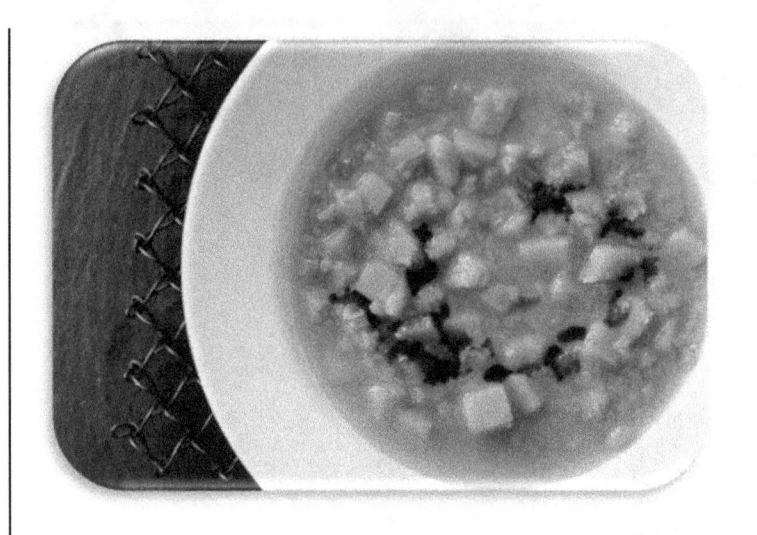

Instructions:

1. In Instant Pot using Sauté function, cook shallots and ginger in oil, uncovered, for 5 minutes, or until shallots are golden, stirring.
2. Add coriander and cardamom; cook 1 minute, stirring.
3. Hit cancel to turn off Sauté function.
4. Add squash, lentils, broth, and ¼ tsp salt to the pot. Cover and lock lid. Select Manual/Pressure Cook and cook at high pressure for 12 minutes.
5. Once cooking is complete, release pressure by using a quick release.
6. Stir in spinach, vinegar, and ½ tsp each of salt and pepper.

Chicken Cacciatore

Prep time: 10 minutes

Cooking time: 25 minutes

Servings: 4

Nutrients per serving:

Carbohydrates – 21 g

Fat – 9 g

Protein – 31 g

Calories – 295

Ingredients:

- 1 8-oz package sliced cremini mushrooms
- 1 Tbsp olive oil
- 1 medium onion, thinly sliced
- 3 cloves garlic, thinly sliced
- 2 Tbsp all-purpose flour
- 1 28-oz can diced tomatoes
- 1¼ tsp dried oregano
- ¼ tsp salt
- ¼ tsp crushed red pepper flakes
- 4 bone-in, skinless chicken thighs (about 8 oz each)
- 1 medium yellow or green bell pepper, thinly sliced
- 3 Tbsp chopped fresh basil or parsley
- 1 tsp balsamic vinegar
- Freshly grated Parmesan cheese, for serving

Instructions:

1. In Instant Pot, select Sauté function and adjust heat to More. Cook mushrooms in oil, uncovered, for 4 minutes.
2. Stir in onion and garlic; cook 4 minutes, or until onions soften.
3. Sprinkle in flour and stir. Then add tomatoes, oregano, salt, and pepper flakes. Stir and scrape up any browned bits on pan bottom.
4. Add chicken thighs, pressing into the sauce. Cover and lock lid. Select Manual/Pressure Cook and cook at high pressure for 9 minutes.
5. Once cooking is complete, release pressure by using a quick release. Transfer chicken to plate. Stir and scrape any bits off the bottom of the pan if needed.
6. Choose Sauté function and adjust heat to More. Stir in bell pepper and cook 4 minutes, or until peppers are just tender. Stir in basil and balsamic vinegar. Serve with grated Parmesan.

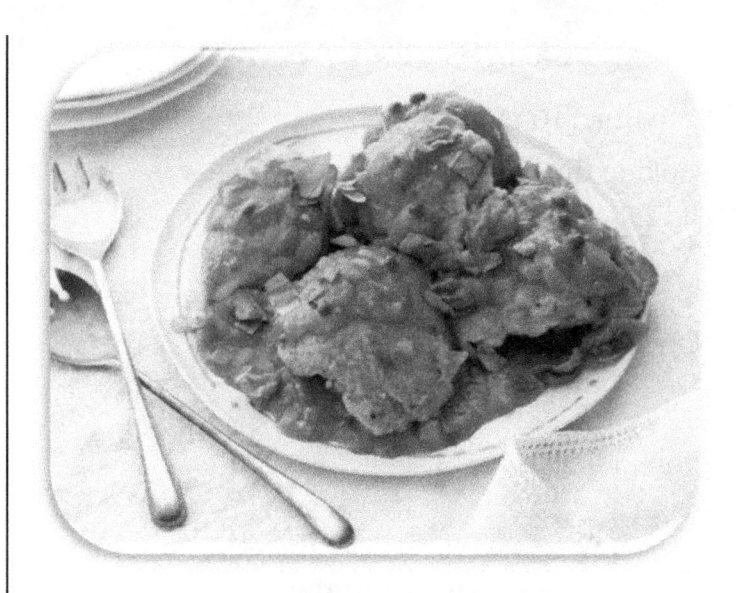

Tex-Mex Beef Sammies

Prep time: 10 minutes

Cooking time: 1 hour 15 minutes

Servings: 12

Nutrients per serving:

Carbohydrates – 30 g

Fat – 21 g

Protein – 22 g

Calories – 420

Ingredients:

- 3 pounds boneless beef chuck roast, trimmed
- 2 Tbsp chili powder
- 1 10-oz can diced tomatoes with green chiles
- 1 4-oz can chopped green chiles
- ½ cup light mayonnaise
- 3 green onions, finely chopped
- 2 Tbsp lime juice
- Sandwich rolls
- Lettuce

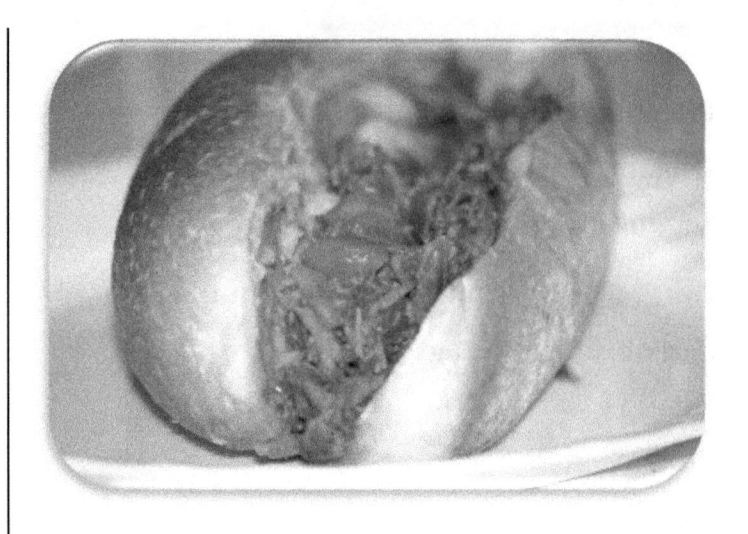

Instructions:

1. Rub beef with chili powder.
2. Pour diced tomatoes into Instant Pot.
3. Add beef and top with green chiles. Cover and lock lid. Select Manual/Pressure Cook and cook at high pressure for 1 hour 15 minutes.
4. Once cooking is complete, release pressure by using a quick release.
5. In a small bowl, combine mayonnaise, green onions, and lime juice.
6. Slice or shred beef, discarding any fat.
7. Serve on sandwich rolls with lettuce and lime mayonnaise.

Apricot-Braised Lamb Shanks

Prep time: 15 minutes

Cooking time: 45 minutes

Servings: 4

Nutrients per serving:

Carbohydrates – 63 g

Fat – 36 g

Protein – 45 g

Calories – 755

Ingredients:

- 4 lamb shanks (about 4 pounds total)
- 1 tsp salt
- ¼ tsp ground black pepper
- 2 Tbsp all-purpose flour
- 2 Tbsp olive oil
- 1 medium onion, chopped
- 1 Tbsp grated peeled fresh ginger
- 2 cloves garlic, crushed with garlic press
- 1 14.5-oz can diced tomatoes
- 3 carrots, cut into 1½-inch chunks
- ½ cup dried apricots
- ½ cup raisins
- ½ cup fresh orange juice
- ¼ cup honey

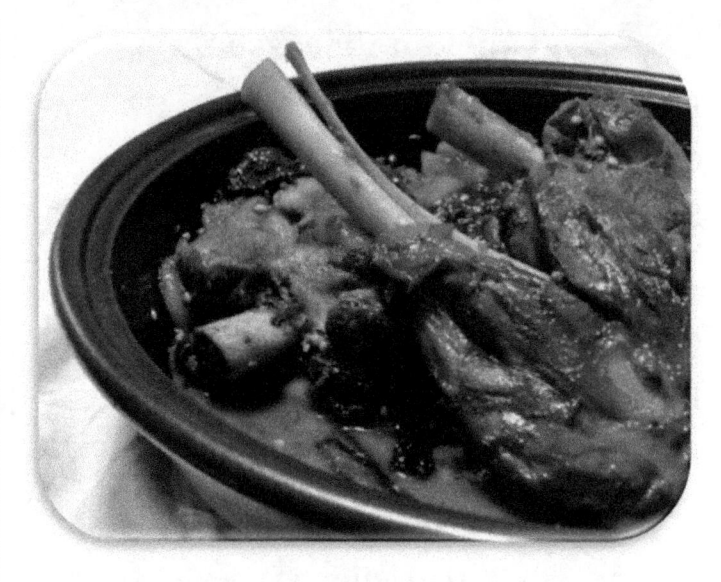

Instructions:

1. Season lamb shanks with ½ tsp salt and ¼ tsp pepper and dredge in flour.
2. In Instant Pot using Sauté function, heat oil. Add shanks, two at a time, and cook 5 minutes per side, or until browned. Transfer to a plate.
3. Add onion to pot and cook 3 minutes, or until softened, stirring occasionally.
4. Stir in ginger and garlic and cook 1 minute. Hit cancel to turn off Sauté function.
5. Return shanks to pot and add tomatoes, carrots, apricots, and raisins.
6. In a cup, stir together orange juice, honey, and remaining ½ tsp salt and ¼ tsp pepper. Pour over shanks. Cover and lock lid. Select Manual/Pressure Cook and cook at high pressure for 35 minutes.
7. Once cooking is complete, release pressure by using natural release function.
8. Serve shanks with pan sauce.

Chicken Fricassee

Prep time: 15 minutes

Cooking time: 45 minutes

Servings: 6

Nutrients per serving:

Carbohydrates – 33 g

Fat – 12 g

Protein – 30 g

Calories – 335

Ingredients:

- 6 large bone-in, skinless chicken thighs (2½ pounds total)
- ½ tsp salt
- ½ tsp ground black pepper
- 2 Tbsp butter
- 2 leeks, white and pale green parts only, halved lengthwise, sliced, and rinsed well
- 3 cloves garlic, crushed with garlic press
- 1 tsp herbes de Provence
- 8 oz white mushrooms, sliced
- 1½ pounds medium red potatoes halved
- 1 cup chicken broth, store-bought or homemade (page 17)
- 1½ cups frozen peas
- ¼ cup light sour cream
- 1 Tbsp all-purpose flour
- Chopped fresh parsley, for garnish

Instructions:

1. Season chicken with ½ tsp salt and ¼ tsp pepper.
2. In Instant Pot using Sauté function, melt 1 Tbsp butter. Add chicken to pot in batches; cook 5 minutes per side, or until browned. Transfer chicken to plate.
3. To pot, add leeks and garlic; cook 2 minutes, stirring.
4. Return chicken to pot. Sprinkle with herbes de Provence. Top with mushrooms and potatoes; add broth. Cover and lock lid. Select Manual/Pressure Cook and cook at high pressure for 12 minutes.
5. Once cooking is complete, release pressure by using a quick release.
6. Transfer potatoes to large bowl. Remove chicken to plate.
7. Add peas to pot and select Sauté function.
8. In a small bowl, whisk ¼ cup sour cream and flour until smooth. Once the liquid in the pot is boiling, stir in sour cream mixture. Simmer 2 minutes, or until thickened. Return chicken to pot.
9. Coarsely mash potatoes. Add remaining 1 Tbsp butter, ¼ cup sour cream, ¼ tsp salt, and ¼ tsp pepper to potatoes; mash. Serve chicken over potatoes and sprinkle with parsley.

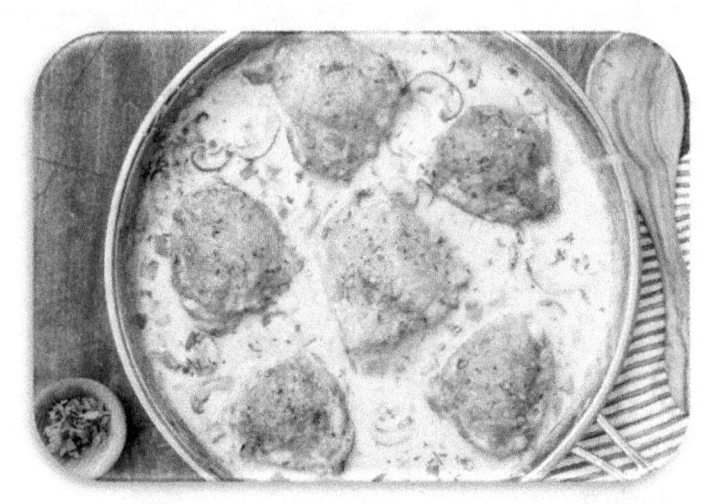

Lemon Garlic Chicken

Prep time: 15 minutes

Cooking time: 30 minutes

Servings: 4

Nutrients per serving:

Carbohydrates – 4.5 g

Fat – 17.5 g

Protein – 66.9 g

Calories – 460

Ingredients:

- 1 Tbsp avocado oil
- 1 onion, diced
- 2 lb chicken breasts
- 5 cloves garlic, minced
- 1 tsp salt
- 1 tsp dried parsley
- ½ cup chicken broth
- ¼ cup white cooking wine
- ¼ tsp paprika
- 1 Tbsp lemon juice
- 3 tsp arrowroot flour

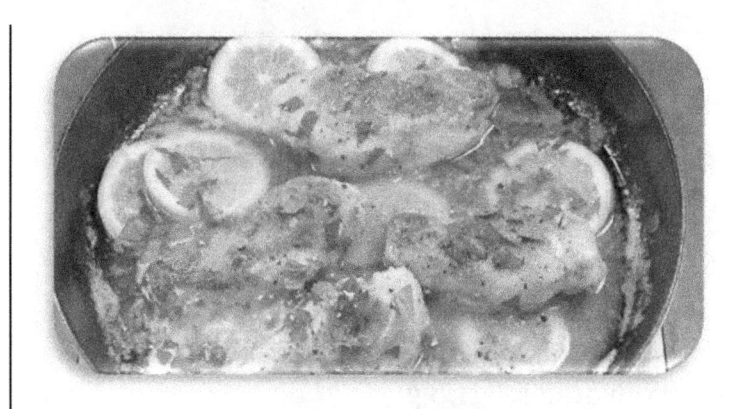

Instructions:

1. Set your Instant Pot to Sauté. Add the avocado oil.
2. Add onions and cook for 5 minutes.
3. Add the rest of the ingredients, except for the flour. Cover the pot. Choose the poultry setting. Cook for 25 minutes. Release the pressure naturally.
4. Take ¼ cup of the cooking liquid from the pot. Add the arrowroot flour to this liquid. Pour it back into the pot. Stir well. Serve while warm.

Spiced Chicken, Chickpeas & Peppers

Prep time: 20 minutes

Cooking time: 20 minutes

Servings: 4

Nutrients per serving:

Carbohydrates – 11.8 g

Fat – 21 g

Protein – 68 g

Calories – 515

Ingredients:

- 1 Tbsp olive oil
- 1 onion, chopped
- 4 cloves garlic, minced
- 2 lb chicken thighs, boneless, fat-trimmed and sliced into medium-sized chunks
- 1 cup tomato sauce
- 2 tomatoes, cut into medium-sized chunks
- 2 red peppers, sliced in half
- ½ tsp red pepper flakes
- 1 can chickpeas
- 1 tsp cumin
- 1 tsp dried parsley
- ½ tsp coriander
- 1 tsp salt
- ½ tsp black pepper

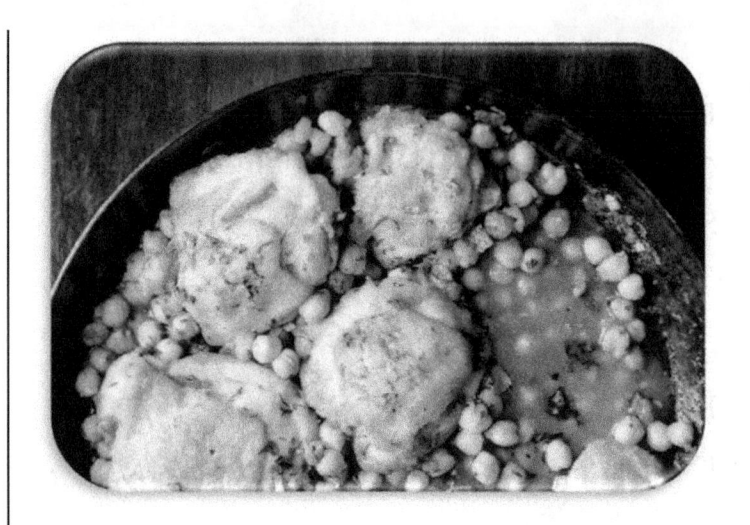

Instructions:

1. Press the Sauté function on your Instant Pot. Add the olive oil. Sauté the onions and garlic for 5 minutes.
2. Add the chicken cubes. Cook for 5 minutes.
3. Add the rest of the ingredients. Seal the pot. Turn to Manual. Cook on low for 10 minutes.
4. Release the pressure naturally. Serve with pita bread or salad.

Chicken in Kale Wraps

Prep time: 15 minutes

Cooking time: 10 minutes

Servings: 4

Nutrients per serving:

Carbohydrates – 34 g

Fat – 14 g

Protein – 29 g

Calories – 370

Ingredients:

- 12 oz chicken breast
- Salt and pepper to taste
- 1 tsp oregano
- 1 tsp rosemary
- 1 cup chicken stock
- 4 Tbsp mayonnaise
- 4 tsp Dijon mustard
- 4 large kale leaves
- 1 onion, sliced into rings
- 1 apple, quarter cut

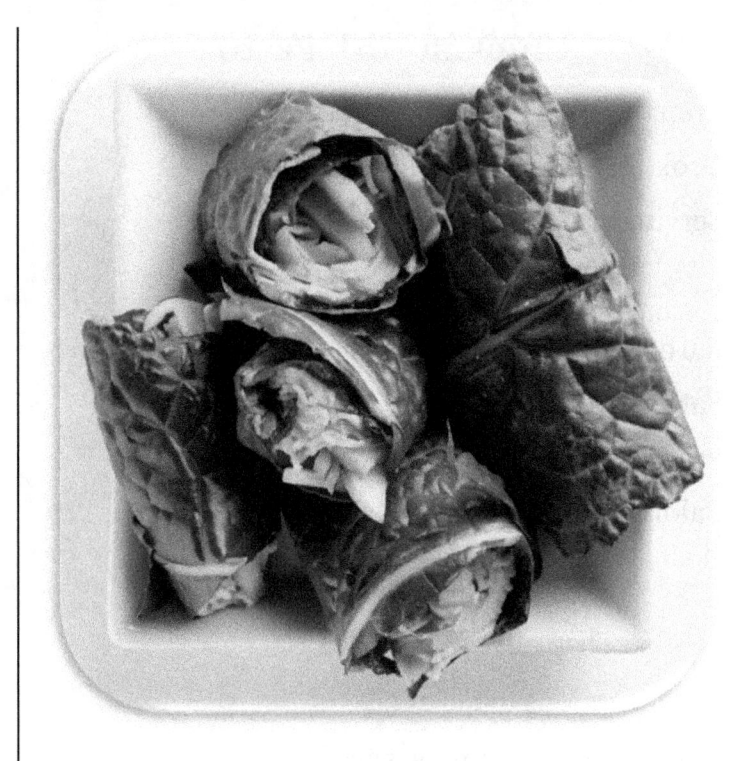

Instructions:

1. Season the chicken breast with the salt, pepper, oregano, and rosemary. Cover the chicken with plastic wrap and marinate in the refrigerator for 30 minutes.
2. Put the chicken inside the Instant Pot. Pour in the chicken stock. Set the pot to Manual and seal. Cook on high for 10 minutes. Release the pressure naturally.
3. Take out the chicken and shred with a fork.
4. In a bowl, combine the mayo and mustard. Spread the combination on the kale leaves.
5. Top each of the kale leaves with the chicken, onion rings, and an apple slice. Roll and secure with a toothpick.

Chicken with Pesto

Prep time: 20 minutes

Cooking time: 20 minutes

Servings: 4

Nutrients per serving:

Carbohydrates – 37 g

Fat – 29 g

Protein – 42 g

Calories – 568

Ingredients:

- 6 Tbsp olive oil, divided
- 2 onions, quarter cut
- 2 yellow peppers, sliced
- 2 zucchini, sliced
- 10 tomatoes, sliced in half
- Salt and pepper to taste
- ½ cup chicken stock
- 4 boneless, skinless chicken breast fillets
- 1 Tbsp green pesto
- 24 black olives, pitted

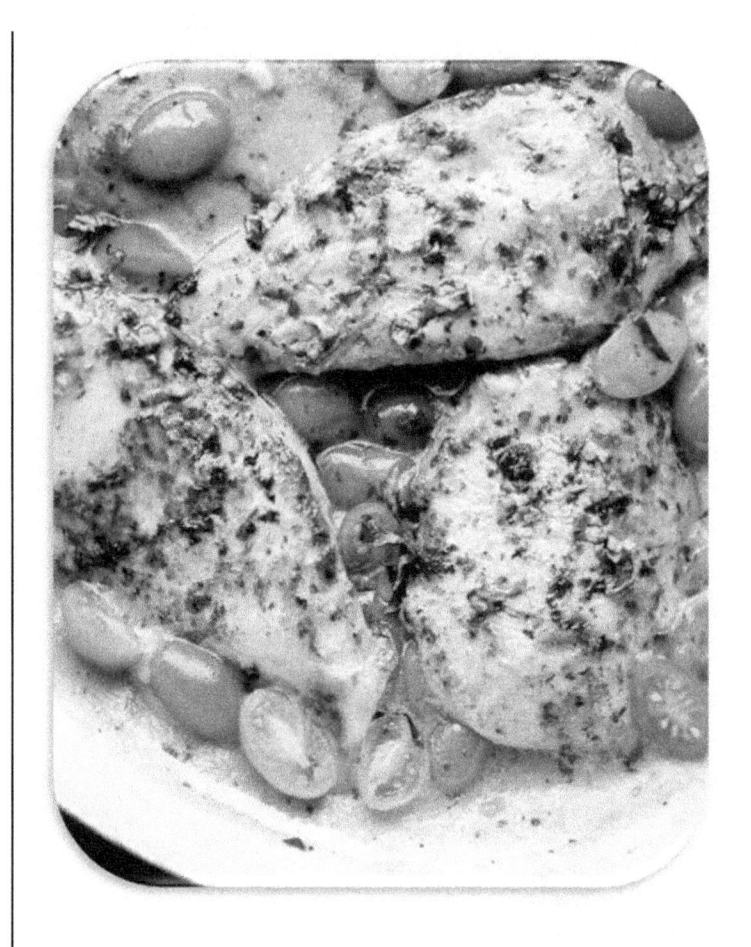

Instructions:

1. Set your Instant Pot to the Sauté mode. Add half of the olive oil, onions, and yellow peppers. Cook for 3 minutes.
2. Add the zucchini and tomatoes. Season with the salt and pepper. Pour in the chicken stock. Simmer until the liquid is reduced.
3. Transfer the vegetables to a platter.
4. Add the remaining oil to the pot. Brown the chicken for 5 minutes.
5. Serve the chicken mixed with the vegetables and pesto.

Beef Casserole

Prep time: 15 minutes
Cooking time: 33 minutes
Servings: 4

Nutrients per serving:

Carbohydrates – 22.5 g

Fat – 17.5 g

Protein – 28.5 g

Calories – 400

Ingredients:

- 2 Tbsp olive oil
- 1 lb stewing steak, cut into cubes
- 2 onions, quarter cut
- 1 yellow pepper, cut into thick strips
- 2 red peppers, quarter cut
- 1 lb ripe tomatoes, quarter cut
- 2 Tbsp sun-dried tomato paste
- 2 oz green olives
- 1 can (2 oz) black olives
- 1 cup water
- 1 cupred wine
- 6 Tbsp fresh oregano, chopped

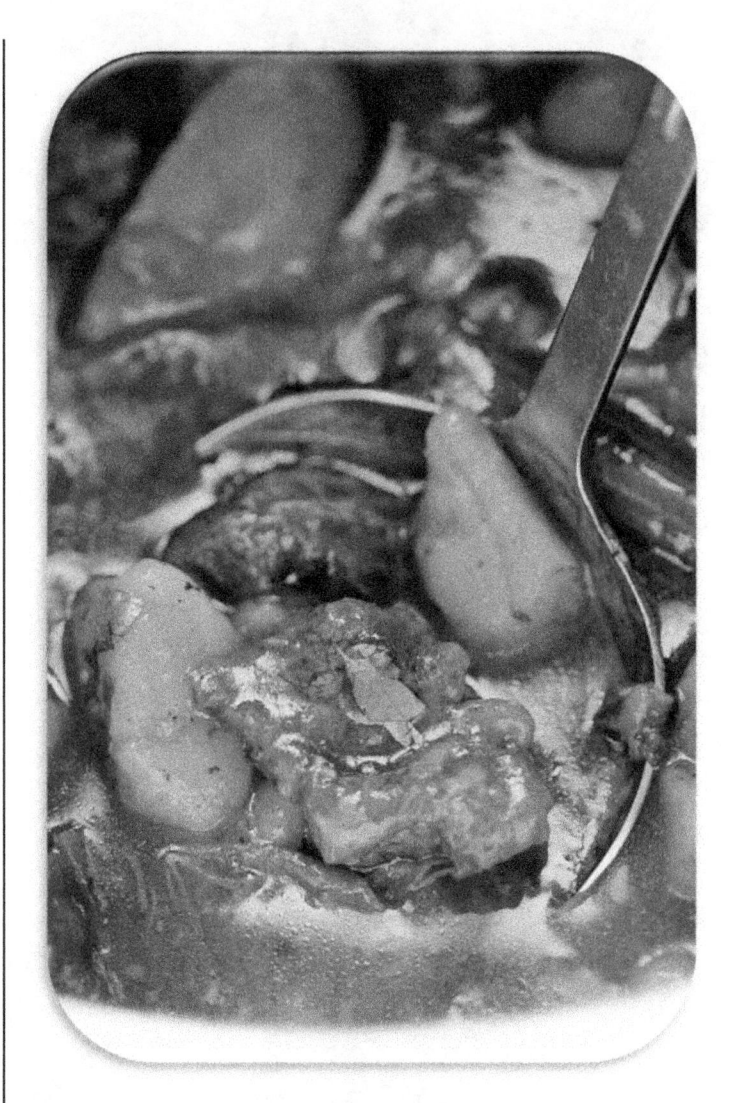

Instructions:

1. Set your Instant Pot to the Sauté mode. Pour the olive oil into the pot. Brown the beef for 5 minutes.
2. Add the onions, yellow peppers, and red peppers. Sauté for 3 minutes.
3. Add the rest of the ingredients, except the fresh oregano. Set the pot to Manual. Cover the pot. Cook on high for 15 minutes.
4. Release the pressure quickly. Garnish with fresh oregano before

Beef with Artichokes

Prep time: 15 minutes

Cooking time: 1 hour 10 minutes

Servings: 4

Nutrients per serving:

Carbohydrates – 26.2 g

Fat – 21.4 g

Protein – 79.7 g

Calories – 616

Ingredients:

- 1 Tbsp olive oil
- 2 lb stewing beef
- 1 onion, diced
- 4 cloves garlic, minced
- 1 14-oz canned diced tomatoes
- 1 15-oz tomato sauce
- 14 oz artichoke hearts, drained and sliced in half
- 32 oz beef broth
- ½ tsp ground cumin
- 1 tsp dried parsley
- 1 tsp dried oregano
- 1 tsp dried basil
- ½ cup Kalamata olives, pitted and chopped
- 1 bay leaf

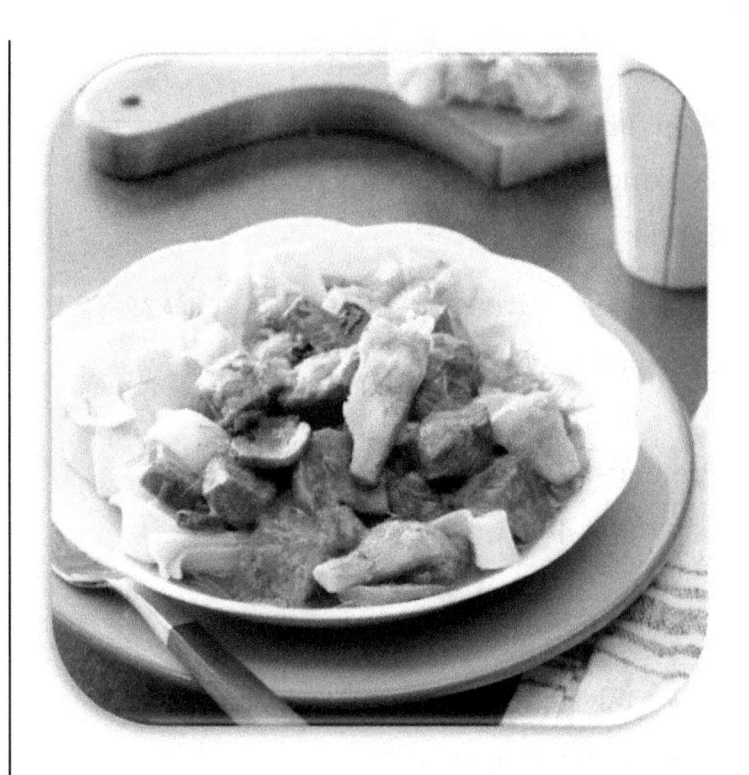

Instructions:

1. Set your Instant Pot to the Sauté mode.
2. Pour the olive oil into the pot. Brown the beef for 2 minutes on each side.
3. Add the rest of the ingredients. Turn the pot to the Manual setting. Seal the pot. Cook on high for 2 hours.
4. Discard the bay leaf before serving.

Beef with Olives & Feta

Prep time: 10 minutes

Cooking time: 1 hour

Servings: 4

Nutrients per serving:

Carbohydrates – 14 g

Fat – 19 g

Protein – 36 g

Calories – 378

Ingredients:

- 2 lb beef stew meat, cubed
- 30 oz spicy diced tomatoes with juice
- ½ cup black olives
- ½ cup green olives
- ½ tsp salt
- ¼ tsp black pepper
- 1 cup feta cheese
- 4 cups cooked rice

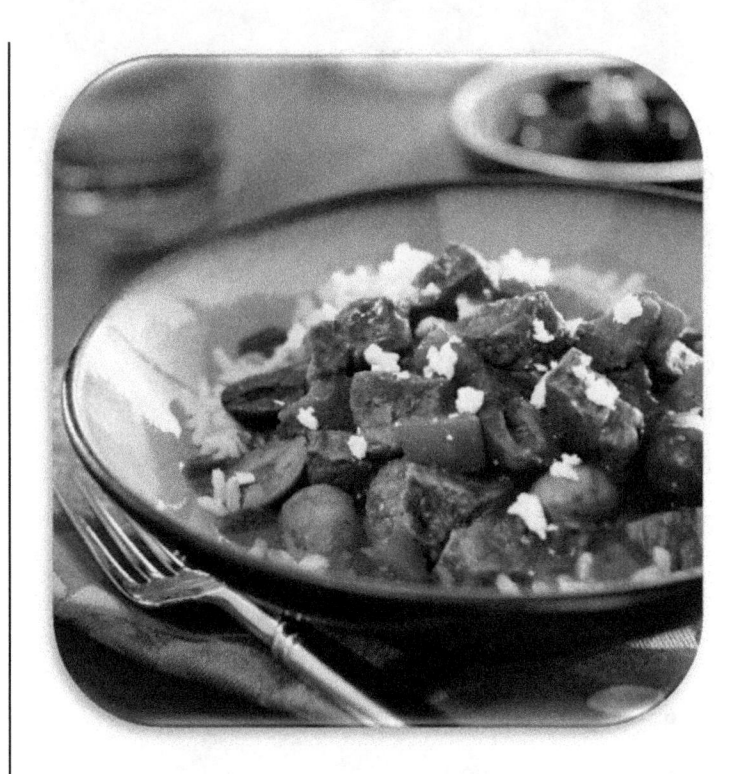

Instructions:

1. Put the beef, tomatoes, black olives and green olives in the Instant Pot. Season with salt and pepper. Seal the pot. Turn to Manual. Cook on high for 1 hour.
2. Top with the feta cheese. Serve with rice.

Beef on Grilled Eggplant

Prep time: 10 minutes

Cooking time: 25 minutes

Servings: 4

Nutrients per serving:

Carbohydrates – 28.5 g

Fat – 24.3 g

Protein – 43 g

Calories – 486

Ingredients:

- 2 eggplants, sliced in half lengthwise
- 2 Tbsp olive oil, divided
- 1 onion, diced
- 2 cloves garlic, minced
- 1 lb ground beef
- 6 tomatoes, diced
- ⅛ tsp salt
- ⅛ tsp pepper
- 1 tsp dried oregano
- 1 Tbsp balsamic vinegar
- ½ cup walnuts, chopped
- 2 tbsp mint

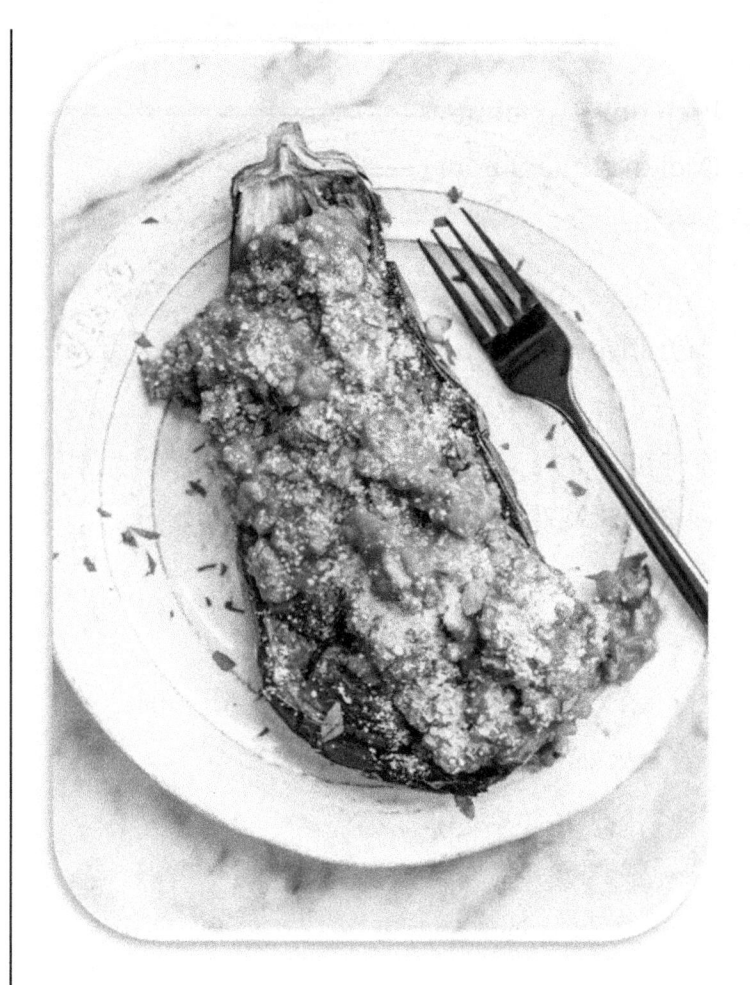

Instructions:

1. Brush the eggplants with olive oil. Grill the eggplants until a little charred. Set aside. Set your Instant Pot to sauté.
2. Pour in the remaining olive oil. Add the onions and garlic. Cook for 5 minutes.
3. Add the ground beef. Cook until brown.
4. Add the tomatoes, salt, pepper, and oregano. Set the pot to Manual. Cook on low for 10 minutes.
5. Top the grilled eggplant with the beef mixture.
6. Drizzle with vinegar and top with the walnuts and mint before serving.

Salmon with Tahini Lemon Sauce

Prep time: 5 minutes

Cooking time: 5 minutes

Servings: 4

Nutrients per serving:

Carbohydrates – 0.9 g

Fat – 20.2 g

Protein – 22.5 g

Calories – 268

Ingredients:

- 1 clove garlic, minced
- ¼ tsp dried oregano
- ¼ cup olive oil
- 1 Tbsp lemon juice
- 1 Tbsp red wine vinegar
- Salt and pepper to taste
- 1 Tbsp feta cheese, crumbled
- 1 cup water
- 1 lb salmon fillets
- 2 sprigs fresh rosemary
- 2 slices lemon

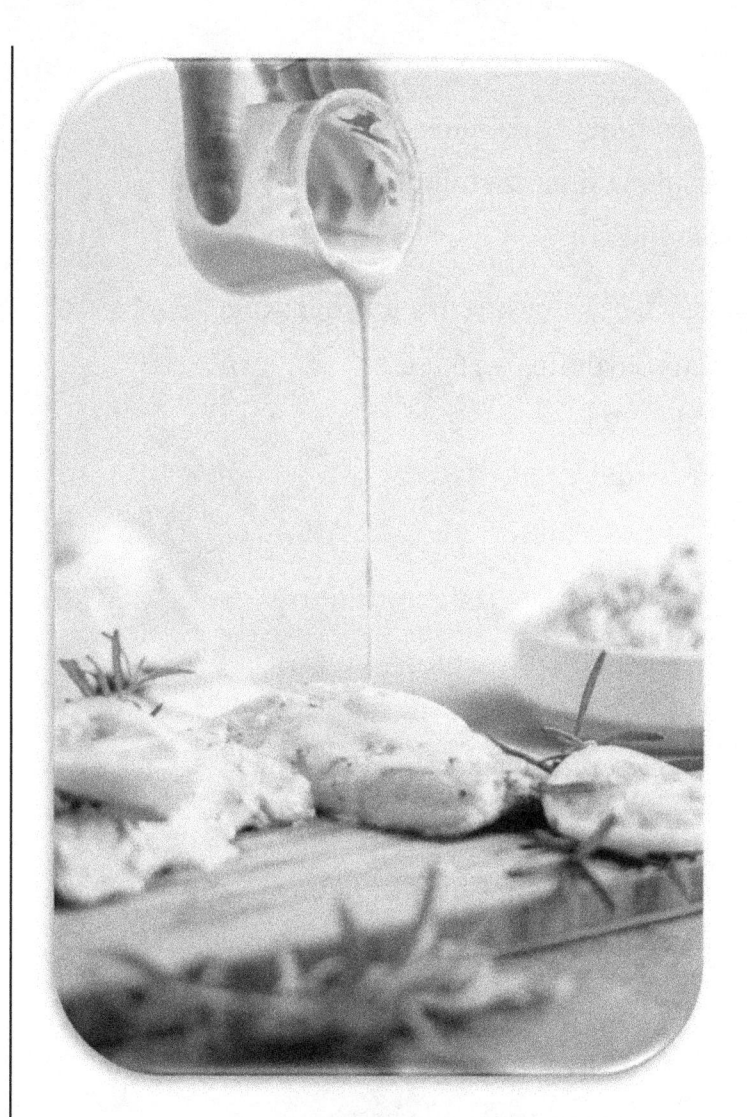

Instructions:

1. Put the garlic, oregano, olive oil, lemon juice, vinegar, salt, pepper, and cheese in a mason jar. Shake for 30 seconds to blend well.
2. Add water to your Instant Pot. Place a steamer inside. Put the salmon on the steamer.
3. Pour the vinegar mixture over the salmon. Top with the rosemary and lemon slices. Lock the pot. Turn it to Manual. Cook on high for 5 minutes. Release the pressure quickly.

Greek Vegetable Soup

Prep time: 20 minutes

Cooking time: 25 minutes

Servings: 4

Nutrients per serving:

Carbohydrates – 76.4 g

Fat – 20 g

Protein – 27.7 g

Calories – 583

Ingredients:

- 3 Tbsp olive oil
- 1 onion, chopped
- 1 clove garlic, minced
- 3 cups cabbage, shredded
- 2 cups cooked chickpeas
- 2 stalks celery, chopped
- 2 carrots, chopped
- 15 oz canned roasted diced tomatoes
- 4 cups vegetable broth
- Salt and pepper, to taste
- ¼ cup crumbled feta cheese
- 2 Tbsp fresh parsley, chopped

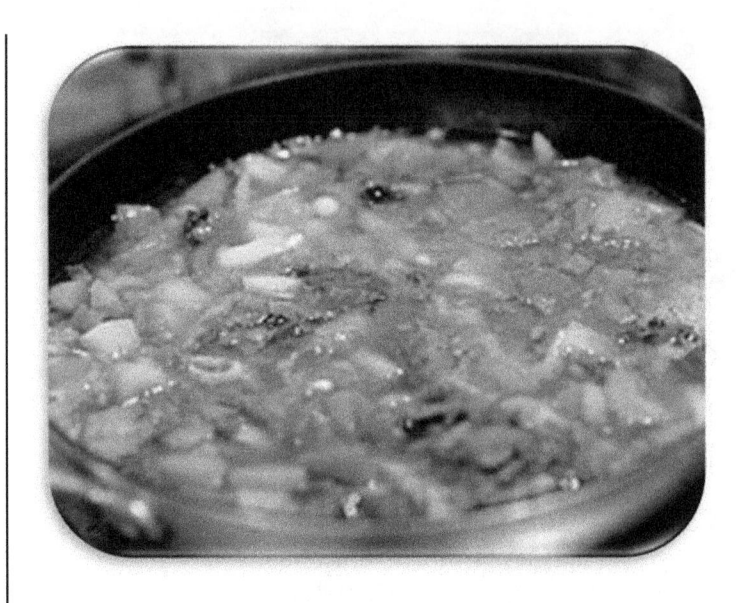

Instructions:

1. Pour the olive oil into the Instant Pot. Set it to Sauté mode. Add the onion and cook for 5 minutes.
2. Add the garlic and cabbage. Cook for 5 more minutes.
3. Add the chickpeas, celery, and carrots. Mix well. Cook for another 5 minutes.
4. Add the tomatoes and broth. Season with the salt and pepper. Cover the pot. Set to soup mode. Cook for 10 minutes. Release the pressure naturally.
5. Garnish with the feta cheese and parsley before serving.

Shrimp, Basil & Spinach Pasta

Prep time: 15 minutes

Cooking time: 9 minutes

Servings: 4

Nutrients per serving:

Carbohydrates – 48 g

Fat – 7 g

Protein – 39 g

Calories – 429

Ingredients:

- 8 oz uncooked angel hair pasta
- 1½ tsp olive oil
- 1½ lbs shrimp, peeled and deveined
- 3 cloves garlic, minced
- Salt and pepper, to taste
- 2 cups chicken broth, divided
- ½ tsp dried basil
- 2 Tbsp lemon juice
- 2 tsp cornstarch
- 4 cups fresh spinach, chopped
- ¼ cup fresh basil, minced
- ½ cup feta cheese, crumbled

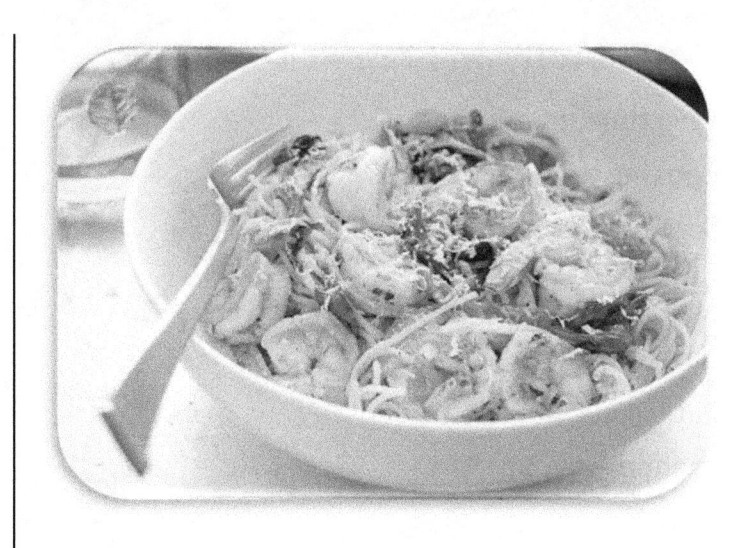

Instructions:

1. Cook the pasta according to package directions. Drain and set aside.
2. Set your Instant Pot to Sauté. Add the olive oil.
3. Cook the shrimp for 3 minutes, stirring occasionally.
4. Add the garlic. Season with the salt and pepper. Cook for 1 minute. Transfer the shrimp to a plate.
5. Add half of the broth, basil, and lemon juice.
6. In a bowl, mix together the remaining broth and cornstarch. Add the cornstarch mixture into the pot. Simmer for 2 minutes.
7. Add the shrimp and spinach. Cook for 3 minutes.
8. Toss the pasta in the shrimp sauce.
9. Top with basil and feta cheese.

Flounder in Stewed Tomatoes

Prep time: 15 minutes

Cooking time: 25 minutes

Servings: 4

Nutrients per serving:

Carbohydrates – 10.3 g

Fat – 7.2 g

Protein – 32.4 g

Calories – 257

Ingredients:

- 1 Tbsp olive oil
- 1 onion, chopped
- 2 cloves garlic, chopped
- ½ sweet red pepper, chopped
- ½ cup white wine
- 14 ½ oz canned stewed tomatoes
- 1 Tbsp capers
- 12 Kalamata olives, pitted and sliced in half
- 1 tbsp lemon juice
- 1 tsp lemon zest
- ½ tsp dried oregano
- ¼ tsp salt
- ⅛ tsp black pepper
- 4 flounder fillets

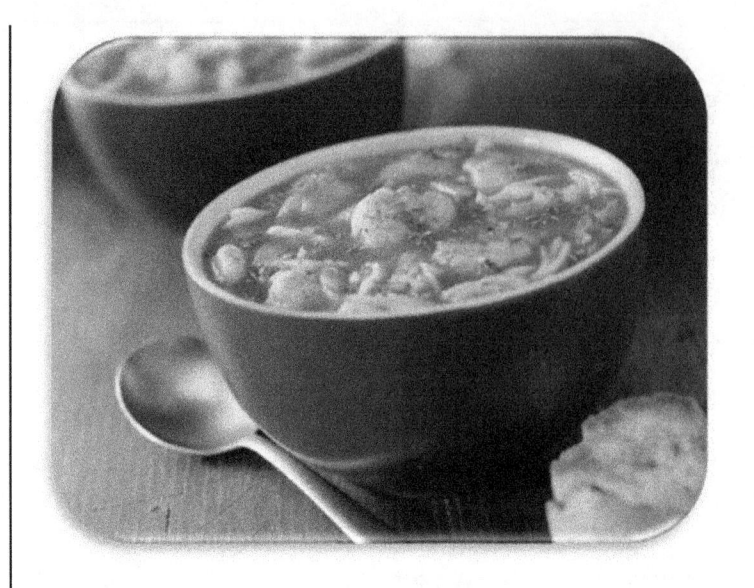

Instructions:

1. Select the Sauté function on your Instant Pot. Add the oil. Cook the onions, garlic, and red peppers for 2 minutes.
2. Add the wine, tomatoes, capers, olives, lemon juice, lemon zest, oregano, salt, and pepper. Simmer for 10 minutes.
3. Add the fish fillet. Cover the pot. Turn it to Manual. Cook on low for 10 minutes.
4. Serve with bread or a green salad.

Tomato & Onion Salad with Tofu

Prep time: 15 minutes

Cooking time: 20 minutes

Servings: 4

Nutrients per serving:

Carbohydrates – 23 g

Fat – 44 g

Protein – 18 g

Calories – 548

Ingredients:

- 16 oz firm tofu, drained and cubed
- 5 Tbsp olive oil, divided
- ¼ cup lemon juice, divided
- 2 Tbsp fresh basil, chopped
- 2 tsp fresh oregano, chopped
- Salt and pepper to taste
- 4 tomatoes, cut into wedges
- 2 cups onion rings
- 1 cup Kalamata olives, sliced
- 2 Tbsp red wine vinegar

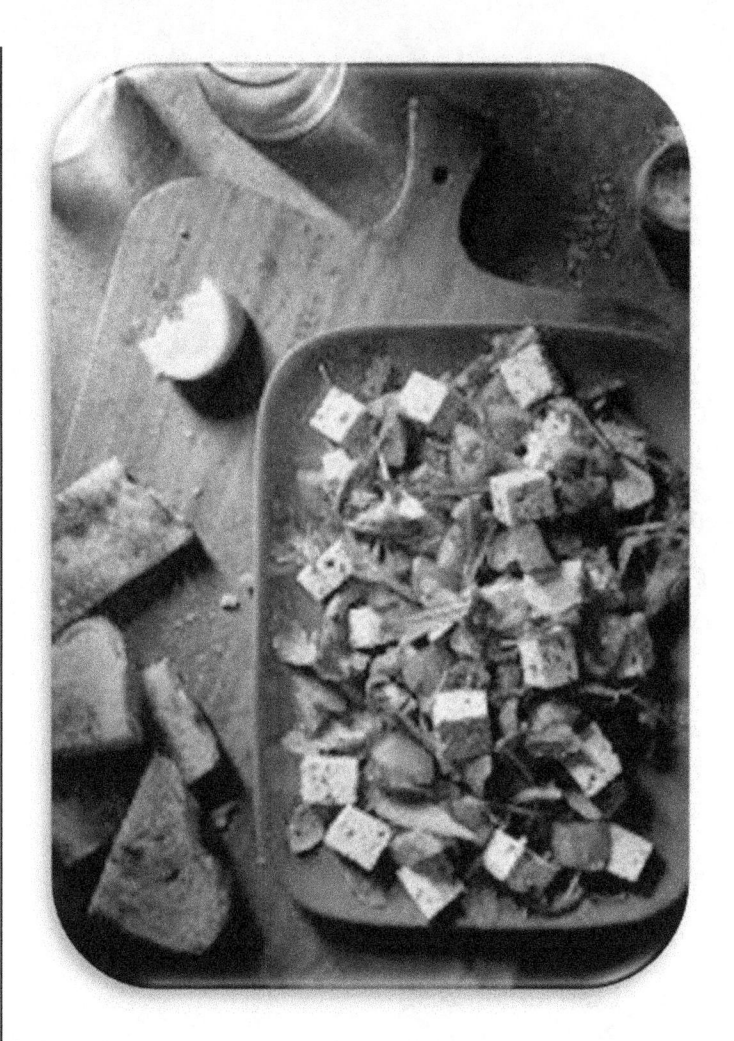

Instructions:

1. In a large bowl, mix lemon juice, basil, oregano, salt, pepper, and half of the olive oil.
2. Soak the tofu cubes in this mixture for 4 hours.
3. Set your Instant Pot to Sauté mode.
4. Brown the tofu for 3 to 5 minutes.
5. In a bowl, mix the tomatoes, onion rings, and olives in red wine vinegar and remaining olive oil.
6. Top the salad with the tofu.

Broccoli in Lemon Garlic Vinaigrette

Prep time: 10 minutes

Cooking time: 5 minutes

Servings: 4

Nutrients per serving:

Carbohydrates – 8 g

Fat – 14 g

Protein – 3 g

Calories – 167

Ingredients:

- 8 oz broccoli, cut into florets
- ½ cup water
- Salt and pepper to taste
- 2 Tbsp olive oil
- 1 Tbsp lemon juice
- 1 tsp lemon zest
- 1 clove garlic, grated

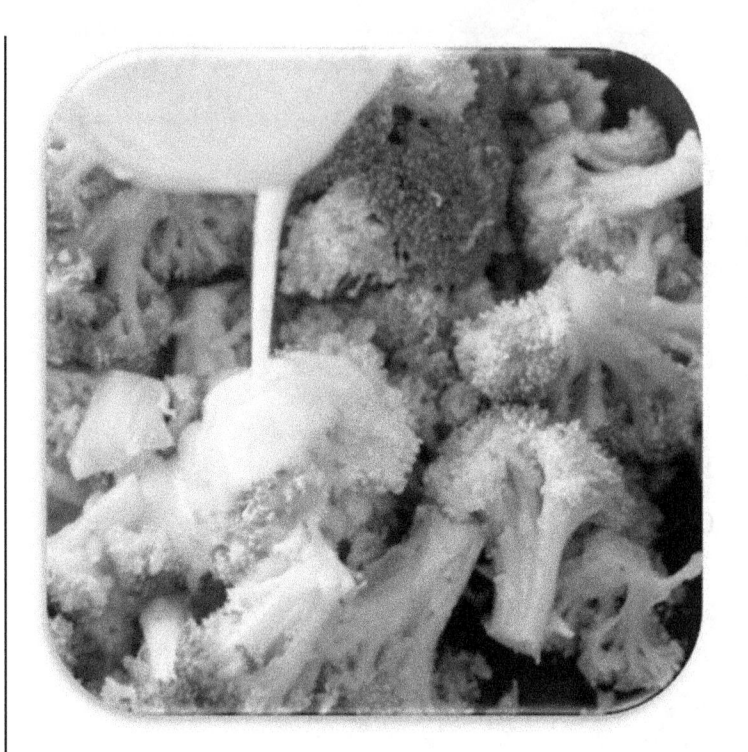

Instructions:

1. Pour the water into your Instant Pot. Put the steamer basket inside. Place the broccoli on top of the steamer basket. Seal the pot. Choose the Manual mode. Cook on high for 5 minutes.
2. Release the pressure quickly. Drain and transfer the broccoli to a plate. Season with the salt and pepper.
3. In a bowl, combine the olive oil, lemon juice, lemon zest, and garlic.
4. Toss the broccoli in the dressing.

Collard Greens with Garlic & Bacon

Prep time: 15 minutes

Cooking time: 30 minutes

Servings: 4

Nutrients per serving:

Carbohydrates – 2.5 g

Fat – 27.3 g

Protein – 26.3 g

Calories – 368

Ingredients:

- 1 Tbsp olive oil
- 4 slices bacon
- 1 clove garlic, peeled and crushed
- 4 cups vegetable broth
- 3 cups collard greens, stems removed and sliced
- 1 jalapeño pepper
- Salt and pepper, to taste
- 1 tsp apple cider vinegar

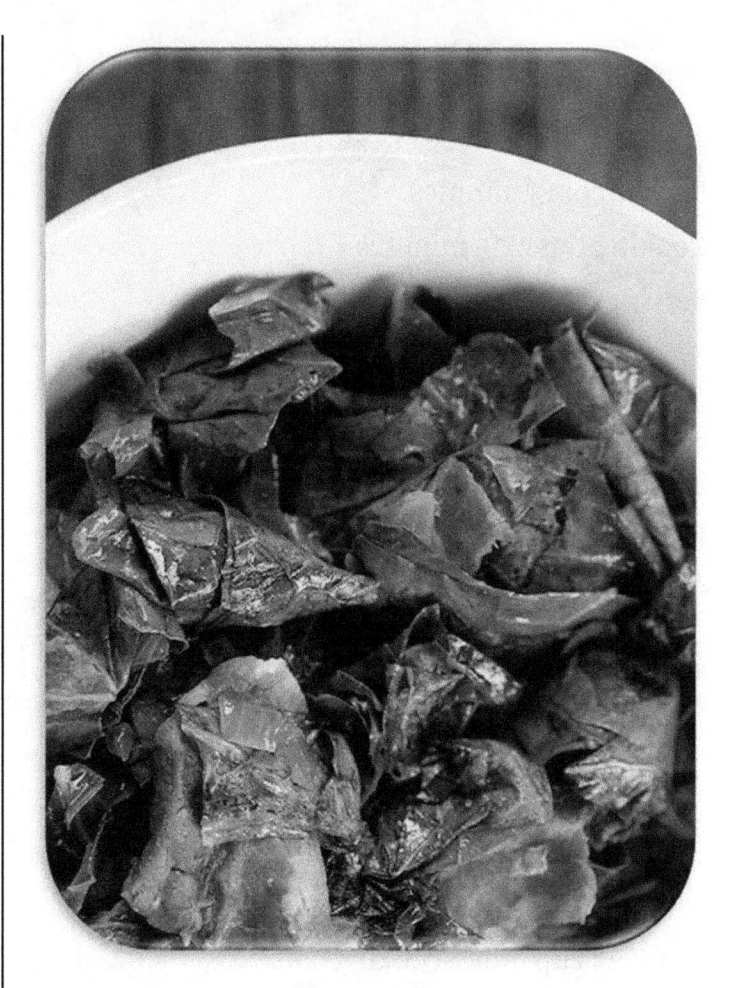

Instructions:

1. Set your Instant Pot to Sauté. Add the olive oil and bacon. Cook until crisp.
2. Remove from the pot. Crumble the bacon and set aside.
3. Add the garlic to the pot. Sauté for 1 minute.
4. Add the broth. Scrape the brown bits from the pot.
5. Add the collard greens, jalapeño pepper, salt, and pepper. Cover the pot. Set it to Manual. Cook on high for 25 minutes. Release the pressure naturally.
6. Top the collard greens with the crumbled bacon. Splash with apple cider vinegar.

DESSERTS

Fresh Apple Crumble

Prep time: 15 minutes

Cooking time: 25 minutes

Servings: 6

Nutrients per serving:

Carbohydrates – 48 g

Fat – 10 g

Protein – 2 g

Calories – 279

Ingredients:

- 5 large apples (about 2 pounds), cut into 1-inch chunks
- ⅓ cup water
- 3 Tbsp 100% white whole-wheat flour
- ¾ cup quick-cooking oats
- ½ cup coconut sugar
- 2 tsp ground cinnamon
- ¼ tsp fine sea salt
- ¼ cup melted coconut oil or butter

Instructions:

1. Add the apples and the water to the Instant Pot and stir well to be sure the apples cover the bottom of the pot in an even layer.
2. In a separate bowl, combine the flour, oats, coconut sugar, cinnamon, and salt and stir well. Add the melted coconut oil and stir until thoroughly mixed.
3. Spoon the oat crumble over the apples as a topping. Select Manual/Pressure. Cook on high pressure for 8 minutes.
4. Let the pressure naturally release for 10 minutes. Remove the lid.
5. Use oven mitts to remove the dish from the Instant Pot and let the crumble cool for 10 minutes before serving warm.

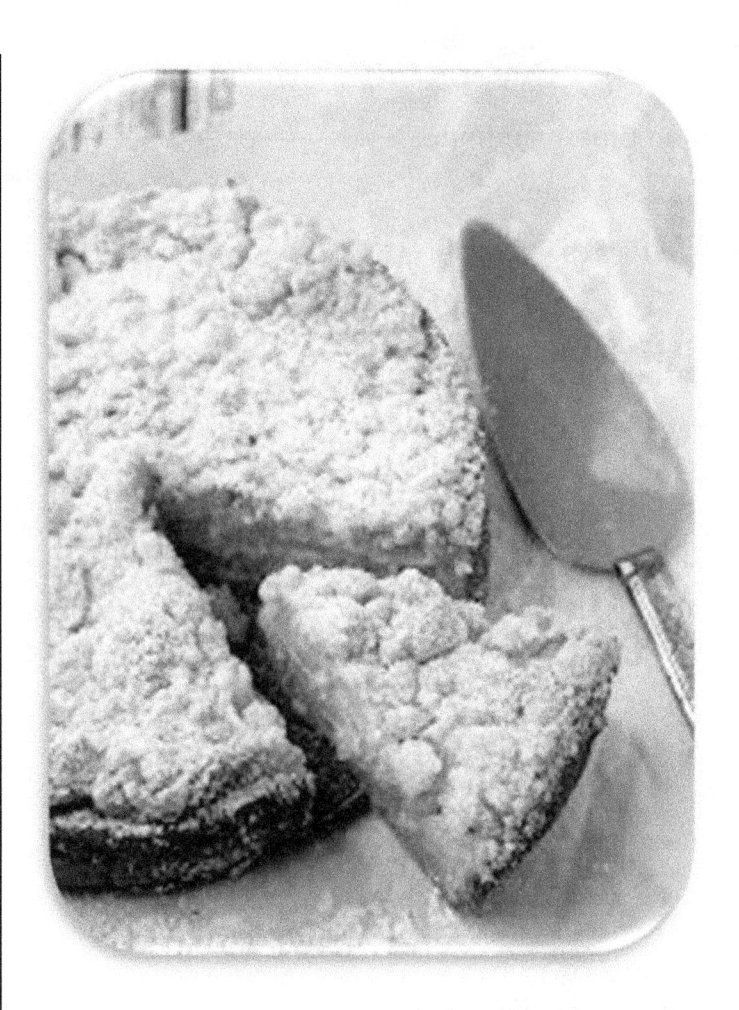

Brown Rice Pudding

Prep time: 5 minutes

Cooking time: 45 minutes

Servings: 6

Nutrients per serving:

Carbohydrates – 39 g

Fat – 12 g

Protein – 3 g

Calories – 260

Ingredients:

- 1 cup long-grain brown rice, like jasmine or basmati, rinsed
- 2 cups water
- 1 15-oz can full-fat coconut milk
- ⅓ cup maple syrup
- ½ tsp pure vanilla extract
- ½ tsp ground cinnamon, plus more for serving
- Pinch of fine sea salt

Instructions:

1. Combine the rice and water in the bottom of the Instant Pot and secure the lid, moving the steam release valve to Sealing. Select Manual to cook on high pressure for 22 minutes.
2. Allow the pressure to naturally release for 10 minutes before moving the steam release valve to Venting. Carefully remove the lid.
3. Stir the rice, making sure that it's tender, then add in the coconut milk, maple syrup, vanilla, cinnamon, and salt. Stir well to combine and adjust any seasoning to taste.
4. Use an immersion blender directly in the pot to briefly pulse the pudding until your desired texture has been reached. The more you blend, the creamier it will be. Serve warm, with extra cinnamon on top. If you'd prefer to serve it cold, transfer it to an airtight container and chill for 2 hours. The pudding will thicken, and you'll need to add water to thin it to your desired serving consistency again.

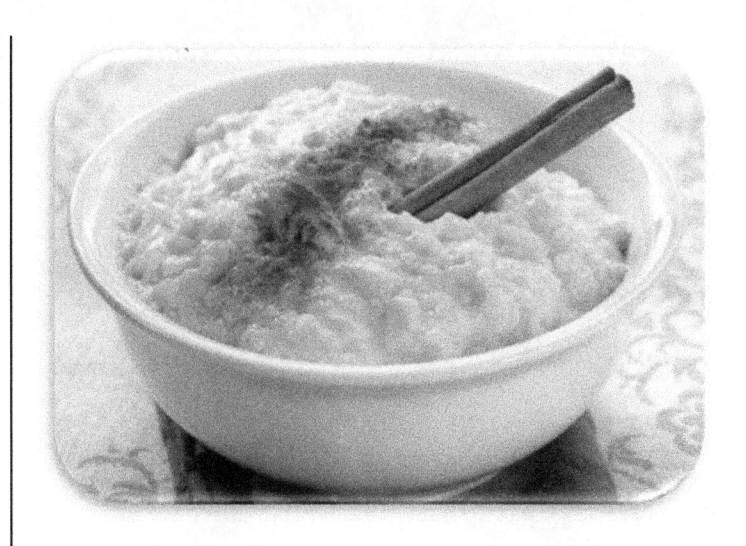

Creamy Coconut-Ginger Pudding

Prep time: 5 minutes

Cooking time: 16 minutes

Servings: 4

Nutrients per serving:

Carbohydrates – 43 g

Fat – 2 g

Protein – 2 g

Calories – 181

Ingredients:

- 1 cup water
- 1 large sweet potato (about 1 pound), peeled and cut into 1-inch pieces
- ½ cup full-fat canned coconut milk
- 6 Tbsp pure maple syrup, plus more as needed
- 1 tsp grated fresh ginger (about ½-inch knob), plus more as needed

Instructions:

1. Add 1 cup water to the Instant Pot and arrange a steamer basket on the bottom.
2. Place the sweet potato pieces in the steamer basket and secure the lid, moving the steam release valve to Sealing. Select Manual/Pressure Cook and cook on high pressure for 10 minutes.
3. When ready, immediately move the steam release valve to Venting to quickly release the steam pressure.
4. Use oven mitts to lift the steamer basket out of the pot and transfer the cooked potatoes to a large bowl.
5. Add the coconut milk, maple syrup, and ginger. Use an immersion blender or potato masher to puree the potatoes into a smooth pudding. Taste and adjust the flavor, adding more ginger or maple syrup as needed.
6. Serve the pudding right away, or chill it in the fridge. Store leftover pudding in an airtight container in the fridge for 1 week.

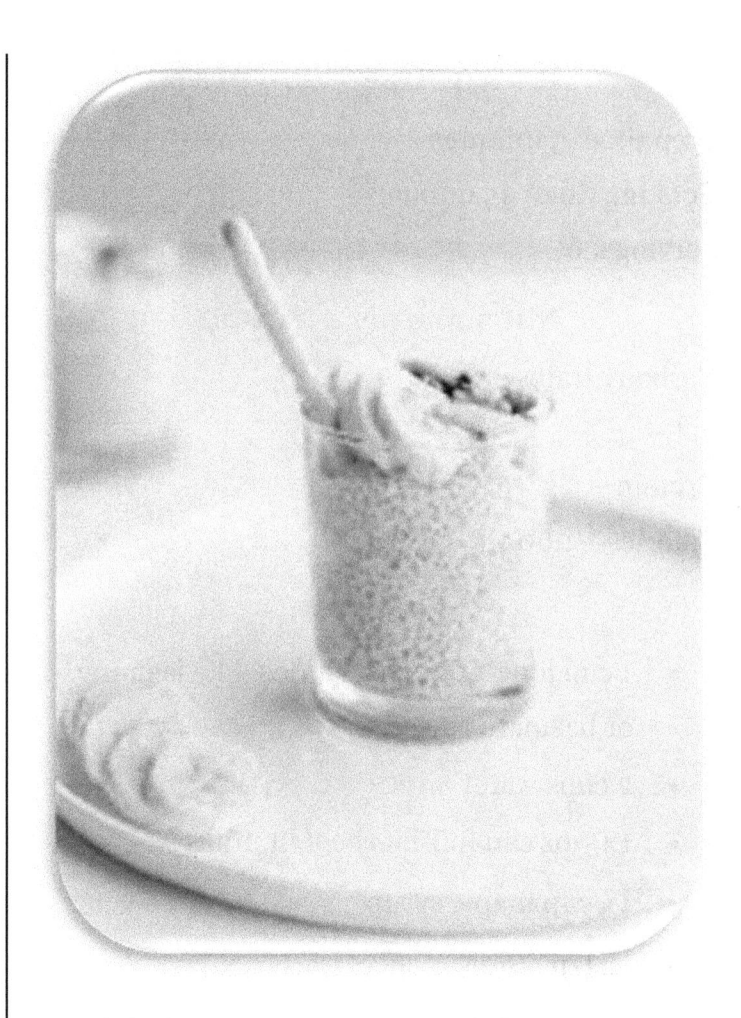

Cinnamon-Spiked Rice Pudding

Prep time: 10 minutes

Cooking time: 30 minutes

Servings: 6

Nutrients per serving:

Carbohydrates – 39 g

Fat – 4 g

Protein – 7 g

Calories – 228

Ingredients:

- 1 cup whole-grain brown rice
- 2 cups whole milk
- Pinch kosher salt
- 1 cinnamon stick
- 1 tsp vanilla extract
- ½ tsp ground cinnamon
- ¼ cup sweetened condensed milk
- ¼ cup raisins

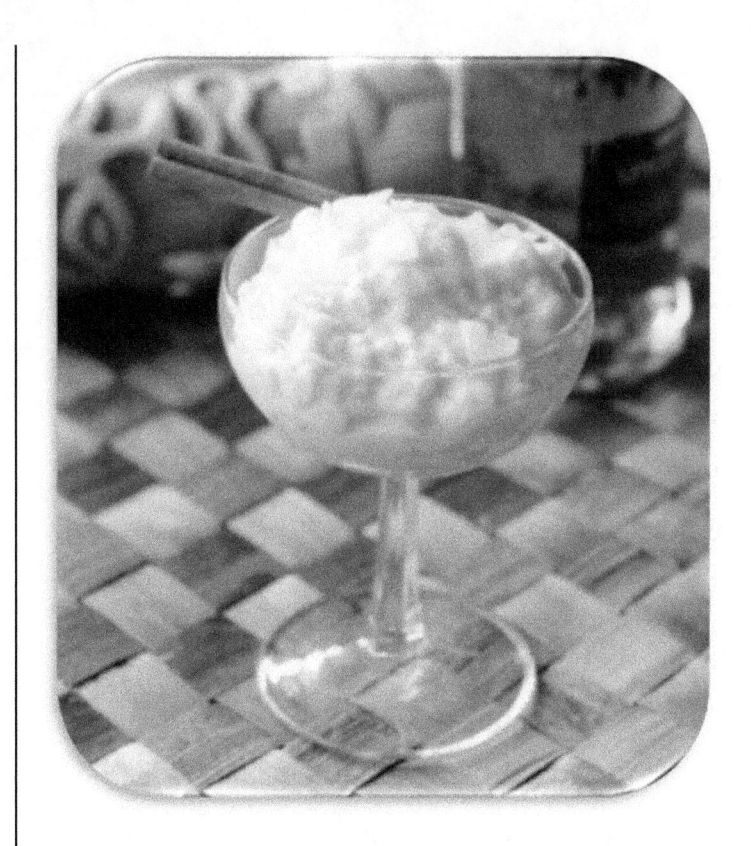

Instructions:

1. Combine the rice, milk, kosher salt, and cinnamon stick in the inner pot.
2. Cover, lock the lid. Select Pressure Cook (High), and set the cook time for 20 minutes.
3. Naturally, release the pressure for 10 minutes, and then quickly release the remaining pressure.
4. Remove the lid. Remove and discard the cinnamon stick, and then add the vanilla, ground cinnamon, condensed milk, and raisins. Stir well.
5. Transfer to serving bowls. Serve warm.

Warm Spiced Cider

Prep time: 5 minutes

Cooking time: 10 minutes

Servings: 8

Nutrients per serving:

Carbohydrates – 28 g

Fat – 12 g

Protein – 0 g

Calories – 120

Ingredients:

- 8 cups apple cider
- 2 cinnamon sticks
- 1 tsp whole cloves
- 1 Tbsp cardamom pods
- 1 lemon, sliced

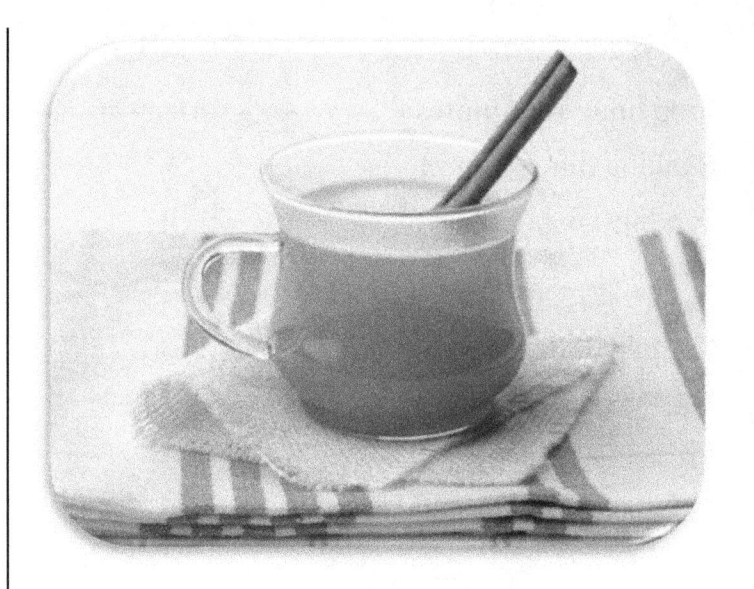

Instructions:

1. Combine all ingredients in the inner pot.
2. Cover, lock the lid. Pressure Cook (High), and set the cook time for 10 minutes. When finished, quick release the pressure.
3. Select Keep Warm, and ladle the cider into mugs for serving. Serve warm.

Poached Cinnamon Pears

Prep time: 10 minutes

Cooking time: 16 minutes

Servings: 4

Nutrients per serving:

Carbohydrates – 36 g

Fat – 0 g

Protein – 1 g

Calories – 150

Ingredients:

- 3 cups 100% apple or white grape juice
- Juice of 1 lemon
- 1 cinnamon stick
- 1 whole star anise
- 3½ cups water
- 4 pears, Anjou or Bartlett

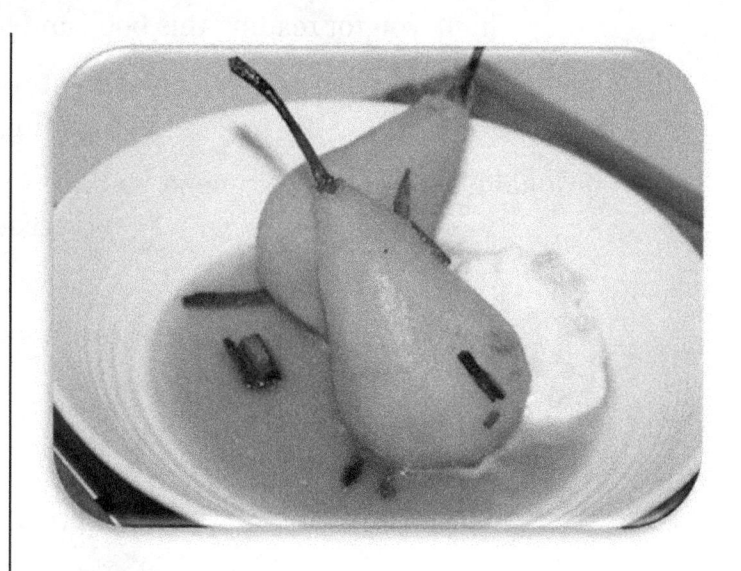

Instructions:

1. Combine the fruit juice, lemon juice, cinnamon stick, star anise, and water in the inner pot.
2. Peel the pears, leaving the stems on. Immediately place the pears in the liquid.
3. Select Pressure Cook (High), and cook for 6 minutes. After finishing, allow the pressure to release naturally, about 10 minutes.
4. Using a slotted spoon, carefully transfer the pears to a serving platter. Serve warm, or transfer the cooled pears to a sealable container and chill in the refrigerator for 3 hours before serving.

CONCLUSION

Thank you for reading this book and having the patience to try the recipes.

I do hope that you have had as much enjoyment reading and experimenting with the meals as I have had writing the book.

If you would like to leave a comment, you can do so at the Order section->Digital orders, in your account.

Stay safe and healthy!

Poached Cinnamon Pears

Prep time: 10 minutes

Cooking time: 16 minutes

Servings: 4

Nutrients per serving:

Carbohydrates – 36 g

Fat – 0 g

Protein – 1 g

Calories – 150

Ingredients:

- 3 cups 100% apple or white grape juice
- Juice of 1 lemon
- 1 cinnamon stick
- 1 whole star anise
- 3½ cups water
- 4 pears, Anjou or Bartlett

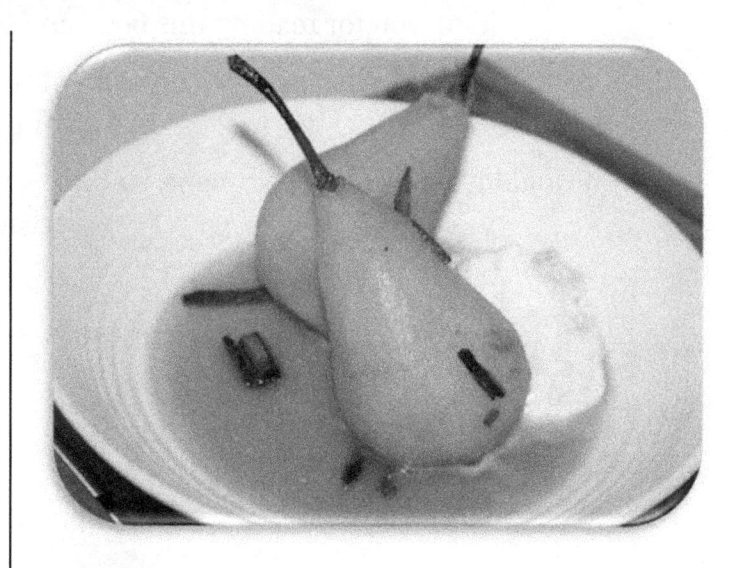

Instructions:

1. Combine the fruit juice, lemon juice, cinnamon stick, star anise, and water in the inner pot.
2. Peel the pears, leaving the stems on. Immediately place the pears in the liquid.
3. Select Pressure Cook (High), and cook for 6 minutes. After finishing, allow the pressure to release naturally, about 10 minutes.
4. Using a slotted spoon, carefully transfer the pears to a serving platter. Serve warm, or transfer the cooled pears to a sealable container and chill in the refrigerator for 3 hours before serving.

CONCLUSION

Thank you for reading this book and having the patience to try the recipes.

I do hope that you have had as much enjoyment reading and experimenting with the meals as I have had writing the book.

If you would like to leave a comment, you can do so at the Order section->Digital orders, in your account.

Stay safe and healthy!

Recipe Index

A
Apricot-Braised Lamb Shanks 43

B
Baby Carrots & Mint..................................37
Basic Bulgur..33
Beef Casserole..49
Beef on Grilled Eggplant 52
Beef with Artichokes................................. 50
Beef with Olives & Feta 51
Broccoli in Lemon Garlic Vinaigrette...............58
Brown Lentils & Spinach Soup.....................24
Brown Rice & Vegetable Pilaf......................32
Brown Rice Pudding 61
Butternut Squash Risotto 31

C
Campfire Baked Beans 25
Chicken Cacciatore 41
Chicken Fricassee 44
Chicken in Kale Wraps 47
Chicken with Pesto 48
Chickpeas & Lentil Salad............................22
Cinnamon-Spiked Rice Pudding 63
Coconut Matcha Quinoa............................. 19
Collard Greens with Garlic & Bacon 59
Coriander Crusted Salmon & Asparagus Salad 26
Cozy Spiced Fruit...................................... 15
Creamy Coconut-Ginger Pudding.................62
Creamy Tomato Soup.................................27

F
Flounder in Stewed Tomatoes......................56
Fresh Apple Crumble................................. 60

G
Greek Vegetable Soup................................54
Green Beans in Mushroom Soup 23

H
Herbed Street Corn 34

Honey-Glazed Carrots.....................................36

I
Indian-Style Lentils....................................29
Instant Strawberry Jam 14

L
Lemon Garlic Chicken................................45
Less-Salt BBQ Baked Beans.......................35
Low-Sugar Pineapple Jam 20

M
Maple Brown Sugar Oatmeal....................... 16

P
Parmesan Garlic Artichokes 38
Parsley & Lemon Chickpeas........................28
Poached Cinnamon Pears 65
Pumpkin Flavored Steel Cut Oats................. 13
Pumpkin Pie Oatmeal 18

R
Risotto Milanese..30

S
Salmon with Tahini Lemon Sauce 53
Shrimp, Basil & Spinach Pasta.....................55
Spiced Chicken, Chickpeas & Peppers.............46
Split Pea Soup with Ham 39
Steel Cut Oats 17

T
Tex-Mex Beef Sammies...............................42
Tomato & Onion Salad with Tofu 57
Tuna Salad... 21

W
Warm Spiced Cider 64
Winter Squash & Lentil Stew.......................40

Conversion Tables

VOLUME EQUIVALENTS (LIQUID)

US STANDARD	US STANDARD (OUNCES)	METRIC
2 tablespoons	1 fl. oz.	30 mL
¼ cup	2 fl. oz.	60 mL
½ cup	4 fl. oz.	120 mL
1 cup	8 fl. oz.	240 mL
1½ cups	12 fl. oz.	355 mL
2 cups or 1 pint	16 fl. oz.	475 mL
4 cups or 1 quart	32 fl. oz.	1 L
1 gallon	128 fl. oz.	4 L

OVEN TEMPERATURES

FAHRENHEIT (°F)	CELSIUS (°C) APPROXIMATE
250 °F	120 °C
300 °F	150 °C
325 °F	165 °C
350 °F	180 °C
375 °F	190 °C
400 °F	200 °C
425 °F	220 °C
450 °F	230 °C

VOLUME EQUIVALENTS (LIQUID)

US STANDARD	METRIC (APPROXIMATE)
1/8 teaspoon	0.5 mL
¼ teaspoon	1 mL
½ teaspoon	2 mL
2/3 teaspoon	4 mL
1 teaspoon	5 mL
1 tablespoon	15 mL
¼ cup	59 mL
1/3 cup	79 mL
½ cup	118 mL
2/3 cup	156 mL
¾ cup	177 mL
1 cup	235 mL
2 cups or 1 pint	475 mL
3 cups	700 mL
4 cups or 1 quart	1 L
½ gallon	2 L
1 gallon	4 L

WEIGHT EQUIVALENTS

US STANDARD	METRIC (APPROXIMATE)
½ ounce	15 g
1 ounce	30 g
2 ounces	60 g
4 ounces	115 g
8 ounces	225 g
12 ounces	340 g
16 ounces or 1 pound	455 g

Other Books by Tiffany Shelton

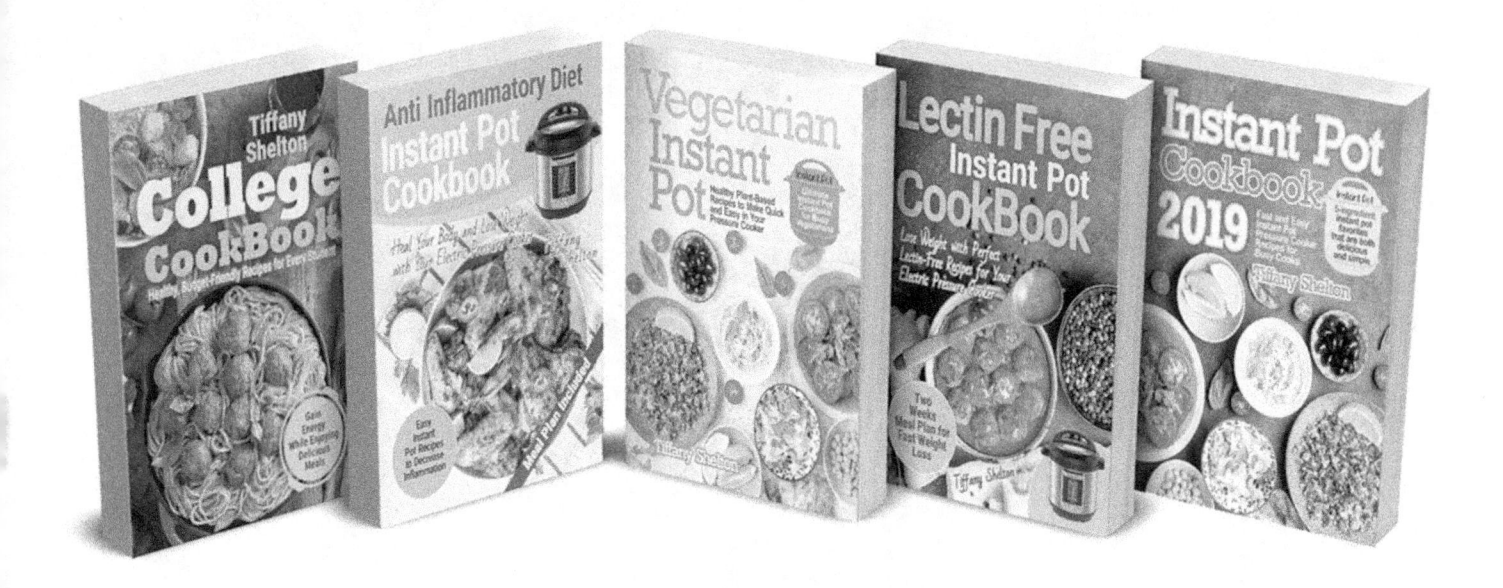

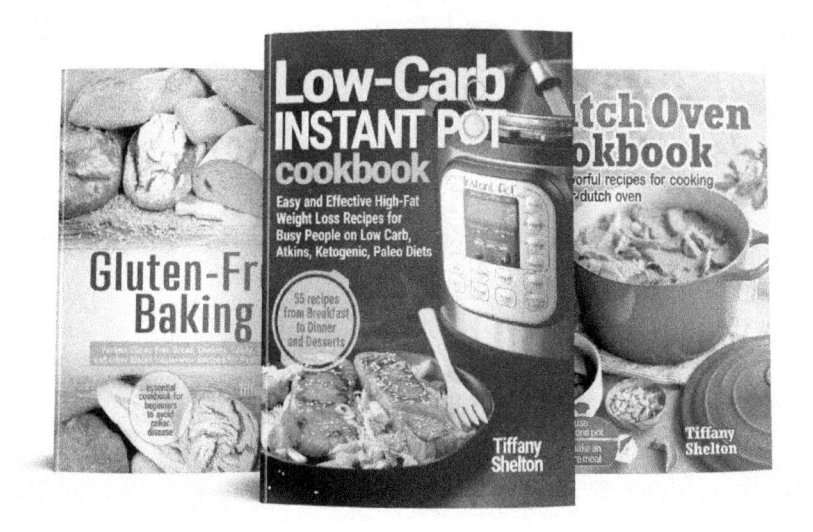

CPSIA information can be obtained
at www.ICGtesting.com
Printed in the USA
BVHW020449300123
657421BV00014B/399